Your Body is Your Teacher

It whispers, until
it has to scream

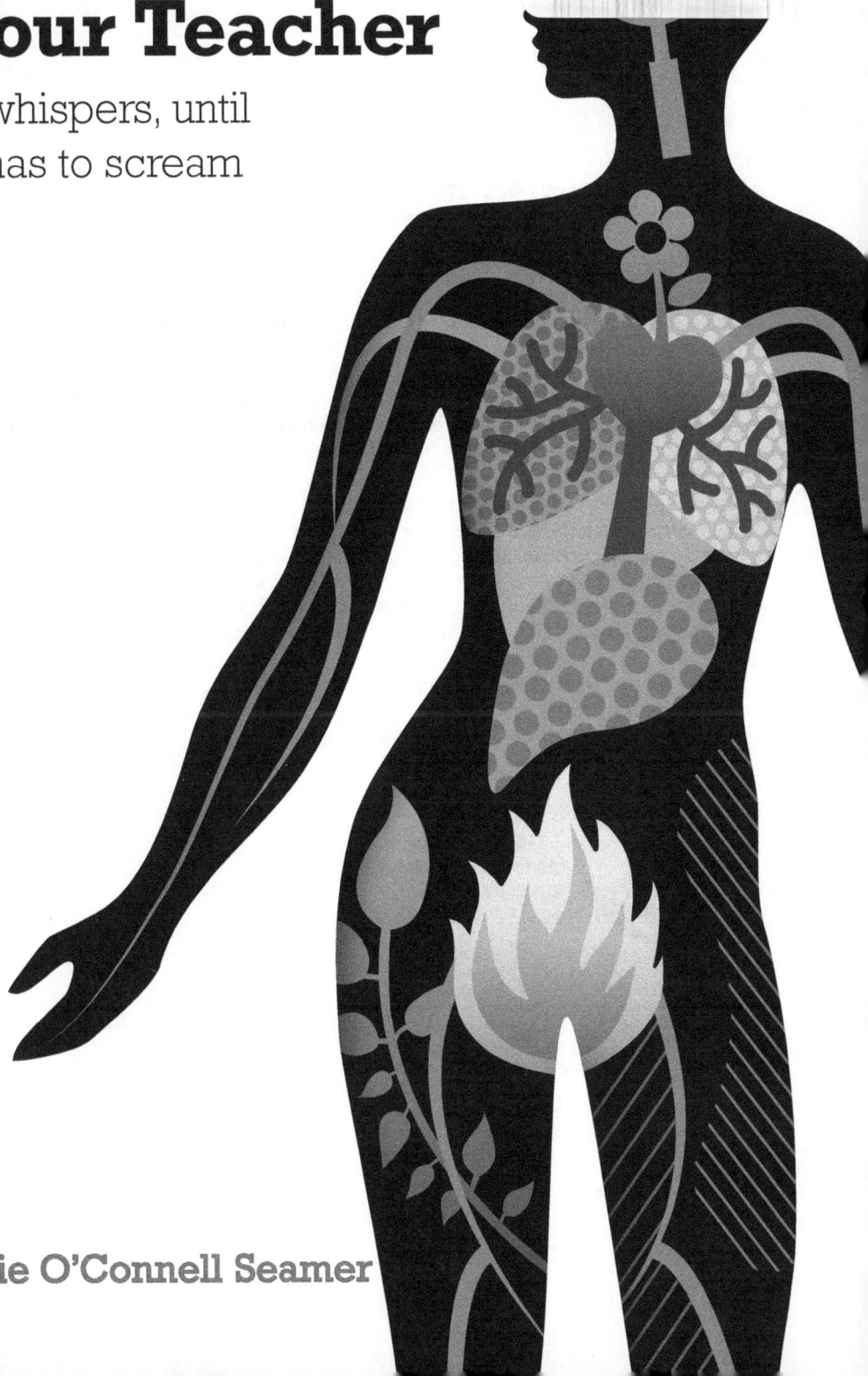

Julie O'Connell Seamer

First published by Busybird Publishing 2019
Copyright © 2019 Julie O'Connell Seamer

ISBN 978-0-6485204-9-8

Cover image: Naina Indira Knoess
Cover design: Naina Indira Knoess
Layout and typesetting: Busybird Publishing

Busybird Publishing
2/118 Para Road
Montmorency, Victoria
Australia 3094
www.busybird.com.au

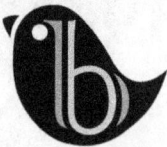

Testimonials

'Julie is very supportive and is not only attuned to an individual's requirements in terms of naturopathy but nurturing in relation to the journey one has been through.'
 – Angela B.

'Julie is a highly skilled Naturopath who takes a functional / integrative approach to healing.'
 – Gareth A.

'As a sufferer of two chronic health conditions, the mental effects were getting to me as much as the physical. At times I felt hopeless. Julie listened to me, she understood my feelings about my struggle. Julie taught me to listen to my body. It screams a lot less now that we communicate better.'
 – Johhny McG

I dedicate this book to my daughter, Kayli Marie.

Darling, I hope you can see that the word
'impossible' is a trick of the mind.

'I'm possible' must be our mantra for life, no matter
the mess, pain, or challenges before us. With self-
belief, our possibilities can unfold.

Contents

Introduction

Life is a process of undoing

*L*etting go is part of the human journey – quitting jobs, relationships, material items or habits that don't serve you anymore. The purpose of undoing is to create space for whatever is both productive and most authentically you – positive sensations, uplifting kinships, useful resources and experiences that bring self-empowerment.

But what if you collected habits, items, thoughts or even ailments that don't serve you, not realising that you're doing so? What if these ingrained attitudes and behaviours have become part of your 'make-up'?

Despite best intentions, of course this can happen. You may walk into my clinic as a prospective client, suffering with ongoing migraines and wanting resolution. You could have experienced these for many years, even decades, and despite trying various treatments (massage, chiropractor, painkillers, etc.) you still can't shake it. You feel tender and irritated. It appears to be a straightforward nuisance that you've grown accustomed to dealing with, but the underlying reasons for this discord remain unresolved. It's begun controlling you. You want freedom from this maddening throbbing in your head. You need to be back in the driver's seat and in control of your own body, but you don't know how to possibly achieve that.

Pharmaceutical efforts can bring a quick fix. They provide temporary control, allowing you to be master of your body again, to push on. There is merit in this; you need to function, after all. But when do these efforts become non-productive or even evasive? Are you shooting the messenger by continually shutting down symptoms that may be trying to disturb you for a deeper reason?

According to Edgar Heim, 'in the course of a fifty-year lifespan, the average adult suffers one life-threatening illness, twenty serious illnesses and around two hundred fairly serious illnesses'.[1] Considering these statistics, it's interesting that we try to rid ourselves of any signs of sickness in our body. Are we avoiding the inevitable?

Our bodies whisper until they have to scream

Ignoring your symptoms can be risky. Sometimes the warning signals of viral infection or other discomforts will dissipate. Symptoms of hay fever can come and go. However, it's been my experience that lasting relief from disease is unlikely to happen unless the deeper drivers to the prevailing condition are discovered and addressed. You may remain captive to the illness and your body will continue whispering, until it has to scream.

Thorwald Dethlefsen in *The Healing Power of Illness* says:

> An enforced change in behaviour is an enforced correction, and is therefore to be taken seriously. But when we are ill, we tend to shy away so strongly from enforced changes in our lifestyle that we generally bring every possible means to bear on making the correction go away … so that we can continue undisturbed along our old, familiar way.[2]

I know for myself that there is some truth in this reluctance to listen, or make change.

Another confounding factor is that we're overwhelmed with choice. Options can create pressure and fear of making the wrong decision.

This can be paralysing, so it's easier to avoid committing in the first place. Psychologists have identified the anxiety we can experience when too many options abound.

There's such a wide range of remedies for every ailment available and access to these options is only a finger click away via the World Wide Web.

With these choices come conflicting stories about the benefits or pitfalls of each. Any wonder we often find ourselves in that common fall-back mode of taking a pill and pushing on, despite possible repercussions to the quick-fix option.

Psychosomatic medicine, the mind–body connection

Further complicating our desire to rank and classify ailments, matching them with a curative outcome, is the arguable influence of thoughts and emotions on health. Think of a hypochondriac who fuels his or her ill health with obsessive and negative beliefs. Or the more modern term of somatic symptom disorder (SSD). This occurs when a person feels extreme anxiety about physical symptoms such as pain; while they're not faking the sensations, their intense thoughts and aversion to falling sick can set off the very symptoms they hope to avoid.

From an outside perspective, it's evident that an obsession with health problems is fuelling their affliction(s). When we consider a placebo effect, where belief drives the physical outcome, we witness how the power of the mind contributes to our wellbeing. This gives rise to the two contrasting perspectives that fascinate me – a mechanistic approach to the body, where the parts and cells define it, versus a vitalistic approach that recognises the inherent energy and meaning in everything, including every organ, down to the smallest particle.

In 1818, Johann Christian August Heinroth first coined the term 'psychosomatic medicine'. Within this framework, symptoms are thought to arise from emotional or mental factors. Unlike conventional medicine, where evidence is relied upon to quantify or provide proof, in a psychosomatic viewpoint there are no illnesses, only sick people.[3] Given we can't exactly 'prove' suffering per se, such an approach surely raises questions – and yet, how we each perceive sickness is relative and will impact how we manifest and experience disease.

The mind–body relationship is at the heart of investigative naturopathy. My intention with clients is to discover the underlying cause of any bodily dysfunction. This may require a referral to another practitioner, such as a counsellor or psychologist. When you actively explore the core disharmony creating your particular 'itch', lasting wellbeing is more achievable. Like Dethlefsen notes, 'Behind every symptom there lies a purpose'.[4] Whether that's true for you or not, a holistic approach will open possibilities of treatment that could bring new solutions and insights. This process may require a personal investment of time. And while a 'soldier on' attitude might seem more appealing, temporary recovery is often not an option for someone who has endured a chronic health condition and wants full, lasting resolution.

When clients present themselves at my clinic, eager to achieve improved wellbeing, I applaud their efforts.

Experience has taught me that insight is gained from professional objectivity. Therefore, I seek help from other experts so I can enjoy the best care for my own health needs. This willingness to invest time and effort is not for everyone, nor is it always needed. My motivation is the recognition that unless we're open to dealing thoroughly with our conditions, the signs of bodily imbalance can eventually make an unwelcome return.

When symptoms wear you down

My late partner suffered from chronic back pain requiring regular cortisone injections. He also endured food sensitivities, which would cause not only a great deal of digestive discomfort, but also serious sleep disturbances. This resulted in an under-current of fatigue, frustration and stress in his life. He was a parent, a full-time working teacher with two extra casual jobs and he was active in social and sporting pursuits; he lived a full and demanding schedule. He couldn't afford to have a bad night's sleep or fail to digest important nutrients needed for his active and demanding routine.

Combined with other outside factors, relentless symptoms were slowly but surely 'breaking' him. Despite trying valiantly to cope – relying on sleeping tablets, anti-inflammatories and painkillers – things weren't improving quickly enough to allow him some reprieve.

My fiancé-to-be committed suicide when I was 21 weeks pregnant with our son. Only 6 months before, he'd announced to friends and family joining us at our joint 40th birthday party that he was the happiest man alive. The morning of the day he died, he kissed my pregnant belly and said to our babe-to-be, 'Dada loves you.' A few hours later he was gone, never to return.

Ongoing depression was a driver to this end result – something that might have been manageable, had the other layers of ill health not developed to crisis point.

Sometimes circumstances get the better of us. Stomach ache that develops into irritable bowel syndrome, for instance, or a sore joint that never fully repaired after a childhood injury and is still affecting your fitness and lifestyle decades later. I avoid making personal judgements about the seriousness of these ailments with my clients, because we all process stress and dysfunction differently. What can be a minor nagging ache for one could be a source of stress and anxiety for another.

Our approach to our symptoms and life plays a part in how we respond and recover from ails. If we're consistently thinking, 'I'm sick of life,' for instance, it's inevitable that sickness will eventually present itself, to match that belief. Then, once we're really feeling physically sick, our negative and unhealthy thoughts or mental habits can be reinforced, setting in place a potentially self-perpetuating cycle that is hard to break.

In terms of our mental wellness, unhealthy habits may become so deeply entrenched that only medication, regular psychotherapy or other unprecedented efforts can assist to slowly rewire our greater body system, for life-changing results. It's important to note here that nutritional deficiencies are typically among the major drivers of disease, even mental illness. So it's less that you aren't strong enough or there's something 'wrong' with your mind and body, and more that you need rebalance and nourishment to reset and recalibrate – and to heal. This *is* possible. But sometimes people don't have that time.

Suicide remains the number one killer of Australian men aged 15–44.[5] Higher in deadliness than the road toll, more lethal than many other known killers. It kills more than eight Australians a day, an average of six men and two women. We're losing our loved ones – young boys and men, and now increasingly young girls and women – to premature, self-inflicted death. I wonder how many of these losses could have been avoided with early intervention and holistic support.

Without a doubt, losing my partner in such an unexpected and tragic way has shaped my view on the importance of mental health awareness in our society. Here was a man who was ashamed of his depression, which might suggest he wasn't coping emotionally and felt out of his depth with life's pressures.

This is a book about life, not death, and how to explore the ways we strive for lasting wellbeing. Our optimal body function is the necessary foundation for this state. Health is wealth – a currency to draw upon.

In my naturopathic practice, the common thread among all clients is the yearning to achieve balance in life; to meet their individual needs while juggling families, work commitments, study and other pressures or goals pulling them in sometimes conflicting directions. Whatever paths we might travel, the one certainty is that our bodies will tell us when things are out of balance and we are blind to our inner needs. And this can be an opportunity for self reflection. However, typically we resist this chance, don't we?

Whenever I've been sick enough that the only solution is to retreat from life and go to bed, I think longingly about my fully functioning body and wish it back again. This reluctance to truly take on board what my body is telling me, to wish the imbalance away, is my default reaction.

Can you relate to this? I make inner deals with the devil (or whomever is holding power over my ails) that I will consume only nourishing food, rest when needed and do whatever is required to achieve wellbeing. I'm desperate to hand over the ransom and get going!

And yet, when the time comes again when my health has returned, after a quick moment of thanks I find myself pushing onward with optimistic self-deception, ignoring my body's little messages. Eventually, I get sick, possibly a repeat of the same condition, and I'm once more bartering with the devil over what I'm prepared to do, to regain health and balance.

When fitness is only 20% matter and 80% mind, it's entirely true that sheer will is a formidable force. Still, our bodies don't lie and for each and every unique being, there'll be a trail of health-related experiences to bring us back in tune with our own innate needs. Whether that involves letting go of stuff that's 'not us' or moving closer to the truth of who we really are, symptoms or ailments can offer a chance for rebalance or recalibration to our essence. And it's in this state that we can truly make a difference to our overall wellness.

I've worked in pharmacies, health food stores, a herbal dispensary, weight loss clinics and operated my own naturopathy consultancy across three states in rural, coastal and city-based areas. In all of these settings, I noticed clients were tired of feeling 'not quite right', and frustrated if symptoms continued to haunt them, despite their earnest quest for health. I know what it's like to have a body not functioning at its best, and feeling unable to fix it. From a position of initial resistance, I've grown to understand how important it is to listen to and learn from my body. I now remind clients that this intuition gives you the power to move toward a fuller experience of wellness. This doesn't depend on being perfect or a health fanatic. It's more about embracing what's happening to your body at any stage of your life, and responding to the signals to develop a holistic approach to recovery and balance.

As you'll read in these pages, there've been moments in my life when ill health presented and persisted; although I didn't realise it at the time, those experiences changed me. Whether it was when you had your tonsils or wisdom teeth removed as a child, or broke a bone as the result of an accident, you've no doubt been through this too, being subtly or profoundly altered in body and mind along your life's journey.

Case studies are included from real circumstances where my clients managed to transform their sense of ill-health to an experience of self-growth. (Their identities has been changed for privacy and confidentiality, but the essence of their case remains the same.) Perhaps these insights will spark a knowing in you too – appreciation for the lessons learned from illness or other times of personal disruption. As Annette Noontil says in her book *The Body is the Barometer to the Soul,* 'I see my body as a vehicle to learn from, not a vehicle to use for sickness'.[6]

While this is easier in theory than in practice, given the endless complexities we present as human beings, it is nonetheless a worthy goal.

1.

What Is Your Skin Telling You?

Nigel was a stay-at-home dad. His wife, a successful lawyer, worked full-time. Nigel had taken on the bulk of the child-rearing responsibilities. A loving father, he arrived in the clinic with their youngest son Max, who had suffered eczema since infancy. The rash had developed into an inflamed bleeding mess that kept the boy awake all hours of the night, scratching and sore. It had been an arduous journey for the family because the itching caused the skin to break further, worsening his pain and irritation.

Nigel himself looked concerned and exhausted. He didn't cut corners in the parenting stakes, attending play groups, doing the extracurricular activity runs and school runs while also maintaining the house and volunteering at the eldest son's Scouts group. They had tried everything over the years to help with Max's skin condition – including lotions, healing baths and removing certain foods out his diet – in an effort to allay possible underlying causes.

Max was feeling anxious about starting at a new school with unsightly eczema that spread across his torso and up his neck.

Nigel wanted Max's skin to improve so his son could be more carefree like his older siblings.

In such cases involving young children, the condition is fuelled less by immediate environmental factors and in great part from inherited factors. Max's mum had been an asthma and eczema sufferer throughout childhood and early adulthood. In terms of the value of testing such causes, whether the new offspring is breast- or bottle-fed, until that child is around five years old the inherited health traits tend to present strongly.

In this case, Max's assessment and full blood examination report showed that markers of inflammation and gastro-intestinal dysbiosis were present. Toxins from his ingested food were being recirculated into his system. Thus, a vicious cycle was occurring: Max wasn't getting the best from his food, and his body was overloaded with an impaired defence system and lethargic lymphatics – the results of which were evident on his skin (arms, hands, neck and torso).

Food allergy is often confused with food intolerance. A food allergy (such as egg, peanut or shellfish allergy) is usually characterised by an immediate and often severe reaction of the immune system to exposure to a specific food. That is, symptoms arise within a few minutes (or up to a couple of hours) of eating or coming into contact with the offending food.

When this exposure occurs, the body makes specific antibodies (Immunoglobulin E, or 'IgE') to 'fight off' the allergens. If consumed again, the body will trigger an immune system response, causing histamine release and other naturally occurring chemicals in the body. Allergic reactions to food can vary considerably in their severity and sometimes can be fatal.[7]

Conversely, in the case of food intolerance, reactions are usually delayed and symptoms may take days to appear. This could range from bloating and feeling unwell to migraine. You may be intolerant to a range of foods that are difficult to identify, given that latent causes can last a long while, with no apparent clear link to what you've eaten. This is why food intolerance is often hard to pinpoint by yourself.

Fortunately, testing for food-specific IgG antibodies is a reasonably quick and easy task for your health practitioner to conduct. This can help remove some of the unknowns, showing which foods have become catalysts for your symptoms. Dr Rodney Ford, who specialises in paediatrics in New Zealand, is a long-devoted food intolerance researcher and believes that 80% of eczema is driven by food intolerance.[8]

Mothers can pass on their own food intolerances to their babies, and evidence is mounting to support that these food intolerances, even if not directly responsible for eczema, are a main driver.[9]

We worked to improve Max's skin and relieve his itching by enhancing gastro-intestinal function and supporting his immune function, with some positive flow-on effects to his ability to sleep uninterrupted. However, the issue still wasn't completely resolved.

At a subsequent consultation, Nigel mentioned that they'd been to a skin specialist who suspected a pork allergy for Max. The family had discounted this because they didn't eat ham and were mostly vegetarian. A thorough and engaged health practitioner will work like a detective: the goal is to put the pieces of the puzzle together, leaving no stone unturned. With Max's parents' consent, we decided to conduct an IgG food intolerance test via a pinprick of blood. This particular test covers 48 common foods that may be causing an intolerance. It indicates whether this sensitivity is mild, moderate or high and the results are evident within 40 minutes.

Despite the family avoiding eating bacon, Max's results did indeed show a high reactivity to pork, surprising us all.

There had to be a cause to this revelation, so we looked at everything included in Max's typical daily regimen. His parents were trying their best to rectify the condition, given it was affecting their son's self-esteem. They were vigilant in giving Max children's chewable fish oil capsules since he was a toddler (the essential fatty acids EPA/DHA being anti-inflammatory in action). They'd bought these in bulk from a friend living overseas, who gave them the parcel on a visit years before.

I wondered what brand and formula these were and after a few phone calls, we'd found a likely solution. The manufacturer confirmed that the capsules he'd long been taking daily were actually pork-derived (others may be bovine or vegetarian). Max had been consuming small amounts of pork gelatine daily over a few years, through the well-intended and caring actions of his unknowing parents, because this detail is rarely shared on ingredient labels. While it wasn't the cause of his eczema, and wouldn't typically be any cause for concern or reactivity (particularly given the very small amount that dose accounted for), the cumulative effect appeared to be affecting Max's skin, among other factors.

By removing these from his diet and including flax seed oil and a kid's liquid fish oil from a local brand, ensuring his digestive system was well supported, things began to change – Max was now able to eat wheat and dairy (which had been previously removed from his diet) and, most importantly to him, rolled oats. Max loved porridge and was thrilled that he could enjoy a hot cereal breakfast again. Moreover, his neck was clear now; no itchiness on the arms or torso either. He was a much calmer boy (as were his parents).

Sometimes, small details and tweaks can have life-changing effects.

Many of us self-prescribe supplements long term, not realising that too much of something isn't always a good thing (even with vitamins!) and can have the opposite effect. Everything we ingest ought to be regulated according to our individual physiology. When nutritional intake is not balanced, illness occurs.[10]

This is why I strongly encourage a dialogue with your pharmacist and doctor, never sourcing supplements from international websites (Australia has strict standards and regulations on therapeutic goods for a reason!) and asking qualified professionals in retail health outlets for guidance, sharing how long you've taken something and why.

Again, these capsules were unlikely to be the cause of eczema, given the strong familial ties, but all factors were accounted for and considered, bringing optimal results. This was a particularly happy outcome, given it wasn't only about achieving clearer skin. After reaching their wit's end in managing Max's condition, the whole family could breathe a sigh of relief with Max feeling so much better, reducing the stress load on them all.

Acne, anxiety and the gut

Without doubt, the skin often reflects what's happening internally. Being the largest organ of our integumentary system and a major eliminatory channel, when we have any toxic overload or are 'holding things in' the skin can display this to our otherwise blind eyes. I've successfully treated people with psoriasis, acne, rosacea and eczema. This can come down to an underlying fungal overgrowth that wasn't apparent to the client. Or it could be the sign of inflammation – a fire that needs cooling and calming, alkalising the body so that restoration can begin.

It's interesting that intestinal alkaline phosphatase (IAP) – 'a superfamily of metalloenzymes' – helps to decrease inflammation in the gastro-intestinal tract. Essential fatty acids (EFAs) have been shown to increase intestinal alkalinity via IAP induction, which explains why supplementing with EFAs helps with cases of inflamed skin. Improving the inner digestive environment enhances the function of outer body systems. These alkalising enzymes are also promoted when a gluten-free diet is followed.[11] This is why a nutritionist may suggest that you reduce your wheat intake if you have a skin allergy.

Acne is a skin condition I'm always keen to work with because the results, once achieved, please sufferers greatly. To this end, I practiced a little while in a high-end skin clinic, helping support women's anti-ageing goals and aiming to restore collagen health.

One of these ladies, Allison, had experienced acne flare-ups that seemed to reflect her life stage. For example, when her relationship with her partner had abruptly ended, her skin was at its worst. On a seasonal level she also struggled most in winter when wearing heavier layers of clothing, not getting her necessary levels of vitamin D and dealing with a more sluggish healing response. Some clients conversely find that summer and hot weather are most aggravating to their skin; for Allison, it was stress, hormones and clothing that spurred on her break-outs. And so by investigating the driver of those processes, we could help support improved health of her skin.

Over a twelve-month treatment period, Allison not only enjoyed clearer, brighter and less irritated skin, but her reproductive cycles also steadied, which meant there were fewer mood spikes to impact the skin again. A healthy win-win scenario was established, instead of one imbalance creating another one.

It's a common occurrence that burnout can change our lives. I find it fascinating then even if you're consuming a quality diet and vigilant about your health, an overload of stress can physiologically change everything. Our neurochemistry affects our gut; for example, stress can cause the opening of otherwise tight junctions between intestinal mucosal cells, thereby inciting leaky gut. The leaky gut will cause gastro-intestinal (GIT) discomfort and possible food sensitivities, with the unaware sufferer enduring a double whammy: mental overload along with stomach issues. If the stress heightens, they could find themselves in a perpetuating cycle of feeling even worse.

Auto-immune disorders are frequently spurred on by major personal breakdowns (the immune system consequently being compromised when stress load is high). Late-onset type 1 diabetes is a condition that I believe can be impacted by exposure to pathogens and subsequent stress, affecting pancreatic function. Whenever a major problem arises in my own life, my digestion switches into overtime and the foods I consume don't metabolise properly. I then experience brain fog and fatigue, creating a cycle of exhaustion and overwhelm. Studies highlight this complex inter-play and how the blood-gut barrier (BGB) regulates not only our moods, nutrient uptake/metabolism, neurotransmitter production and brain function, but also our ultimate long-term wellbeing. The BGB also helps prevent cognitive decline and susceptibility to infection, plus the detrimental effects of endotoxins on our body.[12]

Contemporary evidence

In a published paper 'Acne vulgaris, probiotics and the gut-brain-skin axis – back to the future?', Whitney P Bowe and Alan C Logan teach us that the underlying premise to these links have been long founded.

Over 70 years have passed since dermatologists John H. Stokes and Donald M. Pillsbury first proposed a gastrointestinal mechanism for the overlap between depression, anxiety and skin conditions such as acne. They called this the brain-gut-skin theory, hypothesizing that emotional states might alter normal intestinal microflora, increase intestinal permeability and contribute to systemic inflammation. Among the remedies advocated by Stokes and Pillsbury were Lactobacillus acidophilus cultures. Many aspects of this gut-brain-skin unifying theory have recently been validated. The ability of the gut microbiota and oral probiotics to influence systemic inflammation, oxidative stress, glycaemic control, tissue lipid content and even mood itself, may have important implications in acne.[13]

From my clinical experience, dermatological disorders (including acne) are frequently associated with depression and anxiety. Bowe and Logan identify that:

The mental health impairment scores among acne patients are higher vs. a number of other chronic, non-psychiatric medical conditions, including epilepsy and diabetes. Along with the psychological fallout, there have also been indications that acne patients are at a higher risk for gastrointestinal distress. For example, one study involving over 13,000 adolescents showed that those with acne were more likely to experience gastrointestinal symptoms such as constipation, halitosis, and gastric reflux. In particular, abdominal bloating was 37% more likely to be associated with acne and other seborrheic diseases.[14]

Bowe and Logan go on to note:

In recent years it has been confirmed that hypochlorhydria (low stomach acid) is a significant risk factor for small intestinal bacterial over growth (SIBO).

... SIBO has recently been shown to be associated with increased intestinal permeability. SIBO is strongly associated with depression and anxiety, while eradication of SIBO improves emotional symptoms ... Interestingly, the omega-3 fatty acid-rich cod liver oil advocated by Stokes and Pillsbury may have been ahead of its scientific time. Not only does an omega-3 deficient diet increase SIBO, it has also been linked multiple times to an increased risk of depressive symptoms.[15]

A small series of case reports indicates value of omega-3 fatty acids in both the clinical grade of acne and global aspects of wellbeing.

I've included these insights because it's important to highlight that a modern approach to medicine, in my opinion, cannot be a linear journey. Human beings are complex creatures; our path to healing can involve many intricacies that aren't always simple to unravel. While you may present in clinic suspecting you have a straightforward case of acne or reflux, there can clearly be other factors at play, including the impact of any current pharmaceutical you are taking.

Listening to your body may be step one. Step two may necessitate a willingness to be open, because your condition could be the end result of various other factors.

The heartening aspect is that by exploring and addressing the core source of dysfunction, all aspects of disease will be positively impacted. By working holistically, even if the result isn't absolute resolution, you can at least expect an improved sense of wellbeing, and deeper respect and understanding of the inter-connectedness in your seemingly disparate symptoms.

2.

Stopped By Illness

*I*t was something I'd longed dreamed of achieving: climbing the Annapurna ranges in Nepal. I had read the book *Annapurna: A Woman's Place* by Arlene Blum – the dramatic account of an all-female ascent of Mt Annapurna, the world's tenth-highest mountain and one of the most difficult peaks to climb. It had been the first time Americans had summited the 'mother of the world'.

In Sanskrit, *annapurna* means 'filled or possessed by food'. In the Hindu faith, she is the goddess of food and nourishment. As someone who goes to bed excited about what I'll eat for breakfast the next morning, this all resonated with me. A mountain that meant mother and giver of food … I had to get there!

Apparently, few treks on the globe combine such a vast array of landscapes while bringing you close to the base of 7,000 and 8,000 metre peaks. This is another reason why I chose the Annapurna Base Camp Trek: her terraced rice paddies, lush rhododendron forests and high-altitude landscapes, with Mother Annapurna in view much of the time. It sounded unique and spectacular. I wanted to set foot atop her snow-capped beauty and understand for myself why this classic trek could impact so many others, and be one of the most popular in the Himalayas.

I can still vividly picture the journey, winding slowly but surely up the mountains of Nepal. A suburban girl with a basic backpack, accompanied by another lovely Australian I'd met only a few days before via a notice in a cafe ('travel buddy wanted'). We spent a couple of hours rowing a boat together on Lake Pokhara and decided we could work as a team. So the next day we were in a bus, loaded with chickens and goats and a bunch of locals, setting off into the foothills of the mountains, to begin our trek.

The children were delightful, asking 'pen, pen, pen?' as we came through each village of humble rammed-earth huts and smiling faces. We wound our way upward, as the air got thinner and our anticipation of what was before us grew. I was in my happy place: being active, chasing adventure, meeting new people and loving the great outdoors. We gratefully rested tired legs each night, devoured *momos* (Nepalese dumplings) cooked on kerosene at each camp stop, and dragged our sore bodies further up the endless steps the following morning, sometimes behind a long line of Sherpas, with baskets full of luggage and supplies on their heads. It was meditative and self-assuring to be out in the world, making this goal come to fruition.

Fast-forward only a few months and I'm flat on my back, reluctantly staring at fluorescent lights on the ceiling, wishing I could be anywhere else but here. A nurse arrives at my bedside, folder in hand, diligently working through her checklist. She gives me a sympathetic nod, and tucks the starch sheets tighter around my flaccid legs. I cannot feel them at all from my thighs down. If you were to stick a needle in my skin, I wouldn't even flinch. I'm numb, physically and emotionally.

A note from a governing body for sufferers of this condition that had now become mine:

> During the early part of the illness, especially for the few patients who require intensive care, events can be quite frightening. Most patients were formerly healthy, so that finding themselves suddenly paralysed, helpless, with intravenous lines, a bladder catheter, and a heartbeat monitor that continuously beeps can be emotionally upsetting. If the arms are too weak, even brushing teeth, feeding oneself or scratching an itch can become very frustrating.

> The feeling of utter helplessness, and hopelessness, thoughts of possible death, and the threat of permanent disability, dependence and income loss can be emotionally overwhelming.[16]

The Guillain–Barré Syndrome Association of New South Wales sums up my experience aptly. While I wasn't being intravenously fed, nor did I have a catheter or heartbeat monitor, the fact that my legs could not feel anything, without evident injury, was frightening. I had gone from mountain climber to partially paralysed, and I was terrified of this being permanent. How did it happen and why?

Before arriving in Nepal, I'd been working in Melbourne for a student travel agency. I was in my mid-twenties and this job was helping nurture my travel bug. Around that time, I was also meditating with a spiritual group, attending the regular 5am sessions and enjoying new uplifting experiences of a kind I'd not had before. At one of these sittings, I had a vision of myself hanging washing on a rooftop overlooking the magic and mystical Ganges River in

Varanasi, Uttar Pradesh of Northern India. For a girl who'd never been to India, this image seemed strange. It was a vivid moment and I later wondered why I'd had this vision. Was it prophetic or simply a whimsical unknown longing?

A few weeks later, another one of the international leaders in the group came to our town and I enjoyed her vibrant energy. She drew people to her with her calm, wise, open demeanour. She spoke of an upcoming meditation retreat that was happening back in India and asked if I would be interested in attending, singling me out later to insist I would benefit from the experience. As it happened, the ashram was near the Ganges, so I couldn't help but think there was some synchronicity involved.

However, this opportunity came with a tough decision. I'd have to quit a highly contested job. I loved supporting other young people in their travels and being the person to help facilitate their trips of a lifetime overseas. It was a great industry to work in. And yet it dawned on me that I could explore my desire to climb mountains in Nepal and my love for South East Asia by going to India, so my mind was set.

It was a most enlightening trip. I marvelled at the moment I was hanging my sarong to dry on the rooftop of my hostel by the river Ganges – the vision had played out in real time! Although, looking back, I'm stunned that I managed to survive many crazy moments, including two near-death experiences – a bomb on a train in New Delhi and a bus crash that injured most passengers. These journeys were not for the faint-hearted.

After six months of adventures, I longed for personal space, big skies and fresh air again. I needed to be home among my kindred. My flights had me returning via Thailand, so another round of island hopping seemed fitting and the slower pace was a great relief. However, something was wrong. My body was struggling to hold down any food and a low-grade fever began to escalate.

I'd rented an idyllic treehouse cabin on the top of a small but steep hill, reachable only by a precarious path. It was windswept and wild with the sound of the sea smashing on rocks below. I hadn't timed it very well, as it was also the tail-end of monsoon season; there was water everywhere and impressive tropical storms. This would've been enticing and fun if I weren't entirely alone, and sick. Being a solo traveller, I greatly enjoyed the freedom to do whatever I pleased, but this was one huge downside – being out of contact from others and too frail and feverish to move. I didn't have a mobile phone and the nearest locals were a few hundred metres down the hill.

I was bed-ridden and unable to face the journey out of my shack down the slippery, muddy cliffs. A day passed and another; I was now vomiting violently, unable to hold anything inside me. I began to worry that I might have a serious disease like malaria. In this delirium of ongoing fever, with no help and no way to seek medical support, I started to cry like a child. It felt like an eternity but a few days later, weak and emaciated, I crawled out of the hut and down the rocky hill to the nearest food stall.

I recall trying to nibble a little fruit and plain rice, but my stomach had shrunk so much this was more painful than staying hungry. A few slow sips of soft drink gave me the energy I needed to muster help for my bags to be collected. By the next morning, I'd gotten myself organised for the next transport to Bangkok Airport. I needed to get better, fast. It was frightening to be so unwell and not have ready access to better health care.

On returning safely back to home soil and securing myself a lovely little weatherboard beach house out of town on the coast, my body was still suffering. Not only did the smell of India seem to linger in my skin and lungs, but I was constantly unwell – gastritis, impaired immune function and overwhelming fatigue – and never quite recovering. Maybe I had a tropical disease? I knew it wasn't right to be so sick, and after a few weeks things became worse; I seemed to be returning to my state of delirium that occurred while tucked away in that island hut.

One night after increasingly violent purging, I went to bed weary and determined to seek medical help the next day. But on waking that morning, a strange sensation had hit my entire body, especially my legs. They were numb and heavy, as if I'd been sleeping in the wrong position, stopping the circulation of blood. Frightened, I quickly tried to sit upright in bed and get things moving again. My head was pounding, and I was unable to coordinate my brain and limbs. The sensation of pins and needles stuck into my knees. This wasn't good, and I began to panic because my legs weren't responding at all to my attempts to move. They were totally numb!

Imagine the sight of a woman dragging her body across a road to the shore of a sandy beach. That was me on that fateful day I woke to the numbness in my legs. I was desperate to gain feeling back into my lower half so I literally rolled into the sea, splashing frantically as if the cold water would wake up my bones and muscles.

It wasn't working though. How could this be? Thankfully, my boyfriend was within driving distance and on receiving my frantic call for help, he took us directly to the local doctor's surgery. After a quick assessment the doctor directed that I was to go straight into hospital – he suspected Guillain–Barré syndrome, an autoimmune disorder that affects the extremities of the body. In other words, the immune system attacks the nerves, in the arms and legs at first but possibly travelling upward toward the lungs and heart, in which case it can be fatal. This may have been triggered by dengue fever and gastro-intestinal infection. My nervous system was attacking my defence system – in extreme cases, this process could result in paralysis and disability.

Time passed very slowly, still in hospital, when despair began to set into my mind. I became a living pincushion with daily heparin shots in my stomach to prevent any blood clotting. There were several MRI scans, a few excruciating lumbar punctures and teams of medical students surrounding my bed, curiously engaged in my mystery case. I must've been the worst hospital patient ever, refusing to sit in my wheelchair and attempting to drag my half-numb body up and down the hospital's emergency staircase, trying in vain to make myself stronger, and turning away most meals.

The problem was the paralysis wasn't abating; in fact, it seemed to be increasing, from my shins and knees to thighs. I was starting to panic that it could paralyse my reproductive area and that I'd lose the ability to go to the toilet unaided. I already felt so humiliated and vulnerable.

The elderly lady who shared my room could hardly talk; I wasn't sure what her condition was, but she was moaning all day long until the tranquilisers worked their magic, allowing her to sleep in comfort. Despite the good care, I couldn't help but feel this was a depressing environment, detrimental to my road to recovery.

Everything started to challenge me; the changing shifts of hard-working nurses, the smell of disinfectant, the stiff sheets of my bed, the bright fluorescent lights and the lack of privacy. I wasn't designed to heal in such an environment and couldn't manage to overcome this sensation. I yearned for health and movement and felt there was no way I could possibly improve in my sterile room. While the staff in the hospital were well-meaning and efficient, I was being treated as a lost cause. Back then there were fewer treatment options and it wasn't known how severe my case was, nor how long I might be like this. It took all my personal positivity to stay upbeat and find my own inner strength, believing that I could walk again.

Reading *The Tibetan Book of Living and Dying* was my source of sanity. I was looking for ways to find the jewel within my problem. While I was wary of being melodramatic, the fact remained that I felt weighed down by being partially paralysed with seemingly no lifeline to hold onto.

During a visit by my concerned parents, the severity of the situation sank in. That's the only time in my whole life that I've seen my dad cry, standing awkwardly by my bedside, not knowing how to make things better. I had to get well for my parents' sake and my own. Outside my window that faced a sparkling bay, there were boats sailing by, people walking, swimming and running – and meanwhile I was laying with a nightie, my legs growing flaccid from lack of movement, my body unable to do anything much at all. I was twenty-seven years old and determined that this scenario wasn't going to be the pivotal story of my adult life.

Our cells tune in to our thoughts

Mine was a condition that had no certainties (cause or treatment regimen). Thus, I believed that my only way to tackle it was to control the things I could. For me, lying in bed with endless time on my hands to contemplate life's bigger meanings, I began to wonder where I was stepping towards in life – what was my path? Perhaps this uncertainty was somehow, on a subconscious level, impacting my ability to move forward?

I needed to get out of hospital so that I could control more things again – the kind of food I ate, how I managed my days – and to feel excited and joyful once more, not counting each ward shift change or trying to fend off stray patients who would come to my bedside when I was trying to sleep! I couldn't settle for the answer, 'We're uncertain how long this will affect you, but for now you must remain under strict observation.' Perhaps I needed to be stopped to work out my direction in life?

Given these thoughts, I was surely not about to settle with the status quo. Although there were certain risks, I believed I had to take my healing into my own hands.

In my position, I had little options or control, other than my own sense of positivity. So every day I 'willed' my legs to work again, for my white blood cells to activate the required immune responses, and for this virus or issue to now leave my body. I then imagined myself walking and running freely, sensing the wonderful feel of grass beneath my feet, the blood pumping through my legs. Things working normally again. These thoughts didn't always flow readily; part of me still didn't believe that things would turn out okay, but a bigger part of me knew success in walking again was mostly up to me. My stubborn streak kicked in and I repeated the thoughts of walking over and again in my mind's eye.

It was possibly a radical choice that I swiftly but eagerly discharged myself from hospital. The worry that somebody could stop me or control my freedom to find health in my own way was there, but if anyone dared stop me then they would have really heard about it – I couldn't wheel myself away quick enough!

Coming out, I felt like a prisoner meeting the real world after an age of isolation. Everything sang to me, from the sound of birds to the humdrum noise of a rubbish truck collecting its load. The journey home was one of the happiest car trips I've had. It was remarkable to be back in the land of the living.

The nervousness remained. Still, I would stop myself three times daily – on waking, at noon and again before sleep – to refocus and wish my body to repair itself. With a regimen of herbal medicine, yoga and regular meditation sessions, eventually my limp lower body began responding.

I figured if Olympians can 'see' themselves succeed in their desired outcome, as a vital part of their training, then it might work for me too. I had nothing to lose and was able to focus on myself, given my child-free existence. I've since been witness to the explicit power of our minds, whether in recovery from addiction, injury or seemingly insurmountable grief and loss. And to this day I walk with no trouble, although my lower legs remained a little weak for a few years after the virus. While the doctors claimed this to be a miracle when I later returned to have a final MRI scan, I also know that miracles happen daily: people surviving stage four cancer who have previously been given only weeks to live, families rising from the rubble of devastating bush fires and burnt properties – so many marvels abound.

However, it wasn't only my mindset that drove my recovery. I drew on the virtues of medicinal mushrooms (in a standardised powdered format) and the Chinese herb astragalus.

Traditionally, shiitake mushroom was adopted as a tonic that could relieve the aches, pains and fatigue associated with ageing. It was also used for conditions affecting the heart and lungs, for intestinal worms and for various cancers. Contemporary research has focused on the immunomodulatory role exerted by shiitake mushroom, via the bioactive constituents contained in it – including lentinan (beta glucans), which mobilises the body's own defences against tumorigenesis, infection and other diseases.[17]

Since that time, I've drawn on these virtues to help support clients during their chemotherapy and radiotherapy treatments for cancer. This is only undertaken in conjunction with their oncologist, using clinically trialled formulas with a high safety profile and no observed adverse effect.[18]

Astragalus is also used to 'invigorate vital energy' (qi), and to strengthen bodily resistance to disease. It's commonly prescribed for the treatment of colds, flu, stomach ulcers and diabetes, and is widely used in modern herbal practice in China. Classed as a 'superior herb' in the 2,000 year old classic *Shen Nong Ben Cao Jing*, astragalus has been extensively studied by modern science – particularly for its properties as a powerful immuno-stimulant, coming with a long and enduring history as a potent disease fighter. It's known to increase the count of white blood cells and stimulate the production of antibodies, building up bodily resistance to viruses and bacteria.[19]

This is indeed what I needed to overcome Guillain–Barré, with no looking back.

3.

The Physiological Effects Of Grief

*A*fter the virus/paralysis shock, my life stabilised again. The simple joy of being home and at the helm of my own body was sobering and exhilarating.

I visited my distant great aunt, who is renowned in country Victoria for her remarkable healing remedies and balms, all homemade from wild-crafted herbs. Aunty gave me ideas and inspiration for recovering from illness/imbalance; my confidence in 'getting better' was boosted.

Part of that journey necessitated some changes in direction in my life. Wellbeing and fitness had always been a passion of mine, with health and human relations my star subject at school, so it was unsurprising when I realised that I wanted to change tack and begin a career in herbal medicine and naturopathy.

A great deal of health practitioners love their vocation due to prior experience of being unwell themselves, inspired to share their jewels of wisdom with others. I was in the same boat – disillusioned with media, where I'd been gratefully employed post-university.

Although working in radio had been fun, challenging and highly insightful, and I loved the travel job too, the health industry was calling me.

So I passionately began my qualification, working in heatlh food stores and pharmacies for extra knowledge, loving all that I was learning. Graduating two years later I was ready to help bring bigger meaning to my life's travels, via this vocation.

Given the college was based in Brisbane and seemingly endless clinic hours were necessary, Queensland became my new home. I made the solo road trip northward along the East Coast, packing my belongings for new beginnings. Luckily, I found the perfect job in a herbal dispensary and organics store only a few short days after arriving. I was immersed in making on-the-spot herbal remedies for all sorts of conditions and learnt a great deal in that environment.

There, I also met my future husband and later we moved back to coastal Victoria, where I ran a clinic from home and within two local community health centres. On top of this, I represented a vitamins and supplements brand, conducting iridology sessions and trainings on their behalf all around Melbourne and the state of Victoria. It was at the stage when natural remedies were only just becoming popular in chemists and had yet to go into supermarkets, so pharmacists and their staff had a great need to understand the safe, concomitant use of the various medications and natural products they were starting to stock.

After our daughter was born, we purchased a beautiful property in the Grampians, Western Victoria. It was solar-powered with an acre of organic shiraz wine grapes growing on it. We enjoyed resident emus, wild deer and wallabies on our land, and I relished hiking and climbing the rocky outcrops surrounding us.

Geography and occupation as health predictors

The clinic I worked in was located at the nearest town to our farm, within a bustling compounding pharmacy that was the hub of the rural community near and far. We were in the midst of a long drought; sadly, a great deal of my patients/clients who were second or third generation wheat farmers struggled with depression and risk of suicide, given the dire financial circumstances they were enduring. It was an eye-opener to me, but another realisation crystallised: the significant influence our geography and occupation have on our state of health (or lack of it). I began to see clear patterns in various localities within the state – in the fruit growing belt of Victoria (Shepparton and surrounding region) there seemed to be a great deal of allergies – due, I suspected, to workplace exposure of pesticides used in crop management.

At inner western Geelong, where a small community of Northern Europeans settled over past decades – most of which had their own vegetable gardens and enjoyed homemade meals, soups, broths, and local raised and ethically slaughtered meat – I noticed a much stronger constitution type: healthy limbs, eyes and hearts despite these individuals being well into their senior years. Of course, throughout inner city Melbourne, there were more over-burdened livers to be found, as well as blood–sugar imbalance and adrenal fatigue – 'wired and tired' was the typical scenario for the urban dwellers.

In the case of shift workers, including flight attendants, there appeared to be more hormonal issues from disrupted circadian rhythms and sleep patterns, plus higher rates of infertility compared to other groups I treated. I've since seen studies on how poor sleep from work shifts can increase your risk of neuro-inflammation and post-traumatic stress disorder after a crisis, given sleep is so recuperative and often overlooked in its restorative powers – not only in illness, but also as a preventative to further risk of depression and disease.

We're born with certain predispositions and innate strengths, but when our bodies are exposed to particular external influences, including work and lifestyle choices, these can override or activate particular health outcomes. For example, a person living in a mouldy home can experience aggravated arthritis, which otherwise may not have happened with a supportive diet and drier living conditions.

As a still relatively fresh graduate to naturopathy, these discoveries were fascinating to me, fuelling my desire to help others to be well and stay healthy.

After our daughter's first birthday, due to my husband's work, we sold our yacht brokerage family business in Geelong, and sadly left the Grampians farm behind to move to Sydney. I practiced in a weight-loss clinic where the treatment for all clients was almost identical and, without fail, we achieved the results they wanted.

This wasn't my ideal type of clinical practice because I like variety and challenge, but I could see that we can control factors that seem insurmountable, including stubborn weight gain, debilitating fatigue or rampantly imbalanced hormones. There were a lot of very happy clients at that clinic, although they didn't enjoy those outcomes without committing and stepping up. It was a team effort.

Losing a pregnancy

My career in natural health was thriving by the time Kayli turned two years old – it felt wonderful to have work that was aligned with my beliefs, values, ethics and mission in life.

I was also writing for a nutracueticals company and learning more about the intricate biochemical processes within our body systems. There are always new discoveries in this field of science so I was never short of material to research and share. Going to work was always a pleasure, not a drain.

This impacted me positively; however, my marriage was sadly breaking down, as it had been for a long time, and I was becoming a nervous wreck, despite the joy of supporting clients and seeing them experience life-changing wins in their health and sense of self-confidence.

Not long before this, I had an unknown conception – I was away on a women's hiking trip in the untouched wilderness of southern Tasmania. We flew into our remote location on a tiny airplane and the only way out was a seven-day hike through knee-deep mud! I was in wonderful company and amid nature's wonders, taking my mind off the worries I had back at home.

However, I was carrying a 25 kg backpack up and down mountains, over sand dunes and through boggy valleys. I recall feeling quite nauseous and lacking energy throughout the journey – not typical for me in those circumstances. I usually thrive when pushing my physicality in the great outdoors.

When we finally made it back to civilisation I realised I wasn't in the mood for a celebratory glass of wine and in fact wanted to vomit, even though we hadn't begun eating.

Days later I learnt I was pregnant but was miscarrying, in our bath at home in Sydney. The pain hit me, like labour, and not knowing then that I was losing an early foetus, I tried in vain to relieve the overwhelmingly violent eruptions of my uterus. This experience was sobering. I wasn't in a place to conceive again with my estranged husband. I would've loved a sibling for our daughter but the circumstances weren't right.

I was mourning this loss, the futility of our broken marriage, and many other things. Alarmingly, I ended up bleeding for weeks, giving me ample time to stew over my life and what my body was demonstrating. Doctors later ascertained that I had a couple of cysts on my womb that may have contributed.

During this time, I was relying on a nanny to help me achieve the weekly routine, given Kayli's dad was mostly away interstate and overseas for work. This lifestyle was becoming unsustainable, so with a very heavy heart I packed up our home again and moved back to my home state for family support, leaving him there.

Returning to Melbourne, I joined a sports nutrition company with wonderful working conditions, giving me more financial rewards with lower living expenses and less isolation from extended family. I'd loved the dynamic lifestyle but being in my hometown brought a great sense of grounding and confidence that I really needed. The marital separation and eventual divorce was the hardest thing I'd had to deal with in my life up to that point, especially given the effect it had on our girl Kayli.

Your body hears everything your mind says

I was consumed with guilt and sadness from our family situation, living off nervous energy and losing weight as food was going right through me; my metabolism was accelerated by a nervous stomach and frayed nerves. I probably looked like a normal mum but I was breaking on the inside, crying myself to sleep at night, trying to hold things together to function every day. There just didn't seem to be light at the end of the tunnel.

When our body most needs sustenance, calmness and nurturing, typically these are the times when we turn to fast food, quick fixes, stimulants, and anything that can get us through. Of course, this cycle is unsustainable – if we don't stop to address what is lacking (or in excess) and subsequently worsening our health and longevity, we'll surely be stopped – somehow. For me it was shingles – not only one dose, but two!

This was an excruciating time; my body and face were sore with itchy scabs that looked awful and made me want to keep away from anyone who might see it. My body was depleted, yet over-stimulated. I'd lived on adrenaline for such a long time that I couldn't rest or sleep.

I had to find a way to let go, unravel and get back to stronger foundations. I realised that my body was breaking down, or at least slowing me down to enable this to happen. It wouldn't have been possible otherwise, and because I didn't respond properly the first time I got shingles, the second flare-up forced me to.

It was inevitable that my daughter Kayli contracted the kid's version of shingles (chicken pox) at the same time I was sick; we were both emotionally fragile and needed comfort and support. I was learning that I couldn't function as a single working mum without parenting or mothering myself too, and that this had to begin now.

All our close relationships give us the opportunity to reflect on what's happening within our own lives. Accordingly, family members sometimes teach each other through illness, mirroring any discord that exists within the home. In our case, Kayli and I were sharing symptoms. It makes sense that her emotional stress was mine, and the issues I had with my daughter's father were equally impacting her. We were exchanging the virus between us. To this day, we often bounce off each other like this.

Lost sense of taste and smell

When Pietro sat down, his face was wet with tears. A gentle soul who had risen above family scorn owing to his sexuality, Pietro was still passionately family-oriented, finding his way through his strict catholic upbringing and manhood of his own kind. Pietro was soft-skinned and chubby, which seemed to suit him. However, after much deliberation, and only due to firm encouragement by his housemate, Pietro was seeing me for weight loss support.

Learning what he valued was my objective, because we can draw on these inner drivers to motivate ourselves when trying to rise above old habits. I didn't have to wait long to uncover what was causing the weight gain and how we could potentially turn things around for my new client.

Most disturbingly, Pietro had lost his sense of taste since his grandmother died in his arms the year before. He now had no ability to taste food; even his sense of smell was almost non-existent. Pietro was very close to his grandmother, she being one of the few family members who accepted him for who he was, and it was Pietro's greatest fear to lose their bond. His grief was all-encompassing. He felt empty and void of happiness now she was gone.

To counterbalance this ache Pietro ate frequently, gaining over 20 kg in twelve months. It was this dire feeling of being stuck in his sorrow, and a desire to regain his energy and senses, which led him in desperation to seek a naturopathic consultation – a totally new experience to him, which he quietly doubted would help.

Pietro was still mourning his loss. He was trying in vain to quench his hunger, but sadness had literally taken away his taste for life – his enjoyment and ability to respond to flavours and aromas. We spoke about the possible subconscious factors at play and I referred him to a psychologist and hypnotherapist for counselling to that end.

Physiologically, we focused on improving his metabolism and gut function, immune response and nervous system. The mineral zinc plays a role in taste, so addressing that nutrient deficiency was a focus.

As time went on, Pietro began to register the sensation and tastes of salty and sour. I suggested to him that embracing suppressed emotions such as sadness and anger was a step in the right direction. Yet, his sense of sweetness was still gone, because he felt that there was no happiness in sight.

He'd lost a family member and the woman closest to him, his safety net – subsequently, others' perceived lack of empathy and his sense of loss had effectively shut out his joy for life. If he could work toward restoring those feelings, he may start tasting food again and be less likely to gorge from lack of satisfaction.

Referring again to Dethlefsen, and his take on lost senses:

> The measure in which the sense organs cease to work
> properly is thus the same measure in which ourselves are
> taught to look within, to hear what is going on inside us.
> We are forced to 'reflect upon ourselves' and so to 'come
> to our senses' once more.[20]

Perhaps as Dethlefsen suggests, Pietro's condition was forcing him to review certain emotional influences at play?

As long as Pietro's grief was all-consuming, for him that insatiable hunger couldn't be appeased. Inner emptiness can't be satisfied with food. Once he truly loved and accepted the sweetness of life again, the full spectrum of taste would likely return.

And joyously, it did happen – Pietro not only lost the weight, but later regained his passion for cooking and nourishing his loved ones. As an Italian and lover of food, this was like a rebirth of his truest self, while his grandmother's memory remains close to his heart.

Taste and smell research

Memories of taste and smell experiences are vivid and long lasting, and can play an important role in our enjoyment of life. Together, they accomplish three major purposes: nutrition, protection (helping us to avoid spoiled food and toxic chemicals) and communication (conveying important information to others).

Specialised cells in the human oral cavity can detect at least five basic taste qualities: sweet, sour, bitter, salty, and savoury. Taste cells may also respond to components of fat, calcium, complex carbohydrates and other chemical substances found in foods and beverages. Together with the nose, the oral cavity also plays a role in signalling temperature and touch sensations, and in chemesthesis, a multimodal chemical sensitivity of burning sensations that signals the presence of chemical irritants (such as capsaicin in hot peppers and toxic chemicals in the air). Sensory neurones in the nose can detect a wide array of odours, and the sense of smell plays an important role in the perception of food flavour as well. Each year, people visit a physician for chemosensory problems such as taste and smell disorders, although most of these cases go unreported.

People with smell disorders often have problems appreciating the smell of foods and claim that food is less enjoyable. They may change their eating habits, which may have a long-term impact on overall health. Loss of the sense of smell may also cause a person to add too much sugar or salt to make food taste better. This can be a problem for those with medical conditions such as diabetes or high blood pressure.

Encouragingly, cells that detect chemical signals are constantly renewing and show a remarkable capacity for regeneration. Their locations (in the nose, on the tongue and in the oral cavity) make them susceptible to damage from the environment, so regeneration is required if these cells are to continue to function throughout life. Scientists are interested in learning what enables these tissues to regrow and to re-establish the appropriate connections with the brain.[21]

Grief and the lungs

Pietro's case was fascinating and while, as with many illnesses, I cannot exactly identify where the emotional component influenced the nuts and bolts of his bodily responses, awareness of the connection between emotions and organs is especially strong in traditional Chinese medicine (TCM). In that medical framework, specific emotions have a negative effect on specific organs. Anger is reported to affect the liver, worry or overthinking affecting the spleen, fear the kidneys, and sadness and grief affecting the lungs. In fact, in TCM they don't use the words 'disease' or 'illness'. They say the body is suffering from disharmony; the emotions can be either the cause or the result of the imbalance.[22]

For example, according to the ancient medical texts, the lung is the official organ that receives 'pure qi from the heavens'. Every time we breathe in, we absorb oxygen (pure qi) into our body, before breathing out the waste product, which is carbon dioxide. The lung is our most superficial organ, with its energy circulating just under the skin. Toxic substances are absorbed and eliminated through the skin, and many dermatological conditions such as acne, dermatitis or psoriasis are often treated with lung acupuncture points.[23]

Asthma and emotion

If we turn to more traditional Western studies, a review of the empirical literature on the relationship between asthma and emotion presents an explanatory model of the connection between this lung disorder and feelings. It proposes that asthmatics tend to report and display a high level of negative emotion, and asthma exacerbations have been linked to periods of heightened emotionality.[24]

In Greek, asthma is referred to as 'tight-chestedness'. In Latin, the word for 'tight' is *angustus*, to which the word anxiety is closely related. Perhaps the tightness that is characteristic of asthma does have something to do with fear?

4.

You Don't Need To Be Sick To Get Better

*A*leena is a matronly Turkish woman who enjoys the good things in life. She was referred to me by a fellow practitioner and seemed quite content with herself … 'Just a few niggles to address,' she remarked. Although we're fortunate to have Dr Google at our fingertips to perhaps save ourselves wasted time of unnecessary appointments, there is value in undertaking a professional health assessment to avoid incorrect diagnosis or treatments.

In this case, Aleena felt she didn't have many health complaints, apart from nagging fatigue and some arthritis. Aleena's main focus was to optimise her longevity and feel the best she could for her husband and grandchildren, and to enjoy their sociable lifestyle.

She didn't understand why she felt fatigued, as she was retired. 'Maybe it's just from being a mother to everyone?' Aleena wondered. With seven adult offspring and over ten grandchildren I'd have to agree, given family was Aleena's passionate focus.

When we sit with a health practitioner, we get a chance to be the patient and allow some release of responsibility for all the decisions on whether we're functioning at our best, or not. It also offers a chance to look inside some cracks we haven't realised are potential openings for new ways of being.

In the first session, Aleena didn't offer much personal medical history or greatly detailed information. Her memory was failing and she couldn't recall if anything health-wise had happened in her younger years. My memory isn't always the sharpest, so I could empathise a little with her cloudiness.

However, it gradually came to our awareness, not only in this session but in her subsequent two visits, that there was an element of dysfunction happening for Aleena. She didn't know that having a bowel motion once or twice daily is common practice; hers occurred perhaps once a week and she always had endured gastro-intestinal distention, with terrible discomfort.

What is normal to you may not be considered normal to your neighbour. For Aleena, it was also typical to drink up to fourteen strong Turkish coffees a day. That is, she didn't see her habit as unusual, given her friends and family were also big caffeine enthusiasts. Aleena had a very high acid load impacting her body systems; her joints were suffering from lack of fresh alkalising foods in her diet and taking joint pain management had become a necessary part of her daily life. Her energy had waned so badly Aleena could barely get out of bed until a few espressos released their effect.

Acidity and joint inflammation

In the clinic, I often see a link between a high acid load and inflammatory conditions. If we're experiencing inflammation, it's important to ensure our 'fire extinguishers are working well'. For most of us, we wouldn't know where to start to achieve this.

Conditions like gout and rheumatic arthritis are closely associated with acidity. Optimal body pH levels are the foundation of good health, whereas chronic metabolic acidosis, if left untreated, will work toward the degradation of joints by impeding vital mineral uptake for bone health too.[25]

Moreover, optimal pH in certain bodily tissues/fluid is vital for:

- neutralising stomach acid and aid digestion (gastric juice, bile and pancreas)
- protection against microbial growth (vaginal tissue)
- providing protection against micro-organisms (skin)
- lactic acid levels (muscle, urine, and blood).

When pH is imbalanced, the body will take compensatory mechanisms, many of which will wreak effects further on in life. For instance, abnormalities in acid–base balance may alter immune response, resulting in significant immune dysfunction, or contribute to acidosis of connective tissue in the body, resulting in pain. Interestingly, a study investigating chronic back pain and the use of mineral alkalising supplements resulted in a significant and clinically relevant reduction in pain symptoms.[26]

There are further implications of acidity on our body – metabolic syndrome, diabetes and obesity are all associated with an increased acid load. Given current dietary trends don't favour a healthy intake of alkalising minerals, and our sodium intake has increased by up to 1000% compared to our ancestors, we gain a better picture of why body pH is an important consideration when dealing with chronic lifestyle related conditions.

I gave Aleena a dietary chart to stick on her fridge to help remind her of the kind of foods that would support a healthier acid–base balance. For instance, nightshade foods will often aggravate joint pain after consumption.[27]

During the first year of our irregular sessions, Aleena managed to halve her coffee intake and introduce more alkalising foods into her regimen. Quite a feat! As her body responded to less dehydration, improved sleep, a calmer tummy and more regular bowel motions, Aleena told me that she'd found a new lease of life and started up dance classes – alone! She was a wife who had been always escorted by her husband wherever they went, and as a devoted mother her life was defined more by others' needs than her own. Getting a taxi to our appointments and spending time on herself were very new and exciting changes.

Impressively, Aleena's sharpness of mind improved markedly. She began completing Sudoku puzzles, helping the grandkids with their homework and even started new hobbies – the resultant crafts of which she later sold at local markets. This new financial freedom gave Aleena more impetus to branch out and she left for a cruise holiday with a girlfriend – the first trip in her lifetime that was taken minus her husband's company. This brought a new lease on Aleena's life, which she hadn't been able to imagine as a possibility for herself.

Was this all related to less acidity in her body? Or something else? My sense is that, gradually, Aleena's body systems were being better supported and able to 'fire on all cylinders' again. Each small change she made had a positive ripple effect. And all despite the fact she believed there was 'nothing wrong with her' on initial consultation. The statement that natural therapists help heal not only the symptoms but the whole person counts true here.

It's been many years since our first session together, with return consultations on a twice-yearly basis, Aleena now enjoys only a couple of espressos per day, has healthy daily stool movements and little arthritic pain. Her energy levels are good with the addition of aqua aerobics and belly dancing in her weekly routine. Her sharp mind has allowed her to study a third language and converse with international students who reside in their family home.

Aleena went from a state of advanced ageing to feeling younger than her calendar age. She likes to tell everyone how good she feels. It was almost an accidental recovery – she'd been so busy serving others that Aleena wasn't fully in tune with her own needs prior.

Now she's enjoying optimal wellbeing, proving you can always get better no matter where you start from. I'm still impressed by Aleena's ability to push beyond her initial comfort zone. Although she hadn't allowed herself to listen to her body's messages in entirety, when the time was right her investment into her own needs allowed a revamping of her whole self and her experience of retirement.

If ever I get stuck in a rut, I remind myself how inspired I am by Aleena and her ability to create a richer life for herself, even in later years of life.

The virtue of therapeutic-grade, natural remedies

Certain health fads come and go. Some of these, though, have been administered for medical purposes over centuries. The rhizome of *Curcuma longa* (turmeric) is one example. Dating as far back as 1900 BC, curcumin has been widely used in Ayurvedic medicine for its antioxidant, antiseptic, analgesic, anti-malarial and anti-inflammatory properties.[28] The polyphenols of this herb, known collectively as curcuminoids, are now the focus of clinical trials and have become a household name, available in all forms from your local farmers market, grocery store and pharmacy, beyond the herbalist's dispensary.

Given her initial joint pain, a liquid curcumin preparation was one of Aleena's treatments. Of course, it had further benefits than only anti-inflammatory action for musculoskeletal aspects. Curcumin has proven its virtues with blood–sugar balance, pre- and post-operative use, and in dermatology, ocular health, gastrointestinal health, cardiovascular function and oncology support. I can apply it just as easily to a client with irritable bowel function as I can to somebody with type 2 diabetes or triglyceride and cholesterol level concerns.

The wonder of any herbal approach is the far-reaching benefits beyond the active constituent properties first identified. Herbs are rich in antioxidants and goodness. With Aleena, her nutrient absorption had been compromised due to low stomach acid, despite her imbalanced body pH, making a liquid herbal tonic an ideal part of her improved health regimen.

It's worth noting that many natural therapeutics cross the blood-brain barrier, and this is why turmeric is now well regarded for mental health outcomes, with increasing studies on its applications in depression.[29]

I would suggest that Aleena's overall clarity of mind and improved general wellbeing is attributable to useful natural remedies like this, delivering outcomes beyond the initial desired outcome. Such is the power of natural medicine.

5.

Listening To Our Bodies

During the early years of school, I gladly embraced any chance to skip class and stay home with my mum. She would take me shopping, bake delicious cakes and allow a reprieve from dealing with a certain bully at school who put everyone on edge.

If I ever happened to be unwell, it was an automatic response for me to dramatise things a little, so Mum would take pity and allow me to stay home. Problem being, when I was genuinely sick she would then wonder if I was legitimately unwell, or practicing my acting skills.

I recall her taking me to the medical clinic on many occasions after I complained of back and leg pain along with aches and cramps, making it almost impossible to sleep. Our trusty family doctor would remark, 'Nothing's wrong with her.' The sense of annoyance and injustice when I really did have leg or back pain infuriated me. 'Can't he tell I'm in agony? Why is nobody listening to me?' I would wail.

The aches continued in bed at night, while trying to stand up, and even when I was moving. What was the cause? I was told it was growing pains and to get some rest, as they would eventually dissipate. I interpreted this to mean that nothing could be done, so I sullenly admitted defeat, and learnt to endure them.

I've since learnt that growing pains are indeed real. They typically occur due to increased growth spurts from 8–12 years old. While it appears that few conclusive studies have been undertaken to elucidate the pathogenesis of this common syndrome, certain factors play a part – lowered pain threshold, increased physical activity, reduced uptake of calcium in the bone matrix over a period of time, over-use of limbs and possibility of decreased bone strength. Some research has shown that emotional disturbances are more common in children with 'rapid growth bone pain' and that recurrent abdominal pain, headaches, and limb pains are a group of pain syndromes expressing a reactive pattern to familial emotional disturbances.[30]

After what I perceived to be futile discussions with our doctor, it quietly deflated me that we had no conclusive answers to my discomfort. Sometimes this included sharp pangs of pain in my back, making me double over – or at the other end of the spectrum, long deep aches like my bones had been set in concrete and were aching to break free. Learning to withstand and overcome this sensation was something I simply had to do, given no real resolution or relief was at hand.

When you're young, it's inherent to believe that adults ought to have all the answers. In my childhood, I was learning the gold nugget that trusting your own instinct is an opportunity in honing that intuitive force for use in later years. Unless we trust ourselves as children, how can we cope and function as adults when we're tested frequently by life? Whether it's a decision in parenting or at university or work, our gut instincts are always called upon – crossroads are reached. Which way forward?

With my condition I gradually learnt to stretch more, and rest when my body yearned for stillness. I also had to move when the pain was too great. Going through this and finding my own answers for relief helped me later, during episodes of severe period pain. While the cause was different, ultimately my own response would influence how I was feeling.

Mind over matter – how far can we push?

As a parent, assessing what is true sickness and something constructed is an acquired skill – using that necessary radar which alerts you when to push your child to rise above a sense of frustration or helplessness. Sometimes we must draw a line in the sand.

A former work associate shared a conversation she had with her young teen daughter. Shari had missed almost the whole first term of her first year in secondary college due to stress-induced illness; her education and social life were subsequently suffering, making her feel worse. It was a vicious cycle. The more school Shari missed, the sicker she felt, increasing her anxiousness. She was missing vital time in establishing friendships and finding her way forward in a new school.

Her mother lovingly acknowledged the physicality of her dilemma but also reminded Shari, 'Your mind is powerful, and you are powerful. Yes, you are sick but you also have the ability to overcome this if you really want to.' My reaction to this was, 'Wow – what a strong message to instil in your child!' Giving them the authority and ability to stand firmly in their own shoes and body is a gift that could pay off throughout their lives. Mind over matter isn't always enough, but showing older children like Shari that feeling good is largely in their own hands, that health is relative, may speed the healing process.

Of course, first ensure that their illness isn't only self-created with a general check-up; consider seeking a second opinion to cover all possibilities.

The psychosocial impact of pain

Cindy was a tall, lean nine year old when she sauntered up the stairs to my clinic some years ago. She was accompanied by her grandma Val, who was her primary guardian, owing to the fact Cindy sadly lost her parents to a car accident when she was younger.

Grandma Val said that Cindy presented with prolonged episodes of pain, affecting her sleep and impacting her concentration at school. Fearing the worst, Val had taken her for MRIs and CAT scans – all of which returned with negative results. Val was becoming distraught because the school counsellor and Cindy's class teacher noted that the student's behaviour had become so problematic that a doctor's visit was in order. Going on the feedback from the school counsellor, the doctor had prescribed medication for ADHD (attention deficit hyperactivity disorder). Their suggestion was that Cindy only take the script during school days, not on the weekends.

Attention deficit hyperactivity disorder (ADHD) is a common behavioural disorder diagnosed in children. Development of ADHD is multifactorial, involving genetic, social, nutritional, parental and developmental factors, plus environmental toxins. Needless to say, it's normal for children to have periods of inattention, impulsiveness and hyperactivity.

However, when these behaviours become more frequent, last longer in an episode or become severe, it can affect optimal development. When ADHD is left unrecognised, performance at school will be negatively impacted, potentially placing strain on school and family relationships. For a diagnosis of ADHD to occur, usually a child must have frequent and severe symptoms for at least six months.

In light of these factors, I believe Cindy's diagnosis wouldn't have been made lightly.

General conventional treatment of ADHD involves stimulant and antidepressant medications, combined with behavioural interventions. Stimulant drugs like methylphenidate are commonly prescribed. Interestingly, 20–30% of children don't respond to this drug class and are unable to tolerate them. The most frequent adverse events include anxiety, mood swings, loss of appetite, insomnia and increases in blood pressure and heart rate, with larger dosages potentially contributing to paranoid psychoses.[31]

Cindy was suffering five of these symptoms, along with leg restlessness, which was considered a possible part of her ADHD. Cindy believed she wasn't an ADHD sufferer, so she felt upset and overwhelmed by the prognosis. Unfortunately, these secondary symptoms were fast becoming harder to manage than the initial leg discomfort itself, amplifying the situation. Her agitation became progressively worse, so school was harder to cope with.

I could relate to these kind of pains, having been though my own conundrum with rapid growth and an active lifestyle as a child. So we spoke about the reality of her experience but also discussed whether the medication was actually right for her. On investigating Cindy's pathology tests and obtaining a salivary hormonal profile (via diagnostic testing with a lab), certain key nutrient deficiencies were identified, but not the expected hormonal spikes her grandma had suspected. Overall, here was a healthy young girl, dealing with the emotional impact of physical discomfort. After a couple of subsequent sessions with the school counsellor and a re-visit to her doctor, they decided that she'd been misdiagnosed.

While this seems a terrible mistake to have happened, it's common for the effects of pain to manifest in ways that confound the typical presentation of a condition. For example, in one study, children with musculoskeletal pain were often rated by their parents as having different temperamental and behavioural profiles than healthy normal controls, suggesting a psychosocial contribution to their pain, similar to that seen with other pain syndromes. In other studies, the family environment and psychological distress were also found to contribute to the development of musculoskeletal pain syndromes.[32]

Cindy was managing her feelings of loss from the death of her parents, and living in new circumstances. Vitamin K2 was a key part of her treatment thereafter. It's a useful nutrient for bone pain by helping support the inner bone matrix during cell turnover.

> Bone is a dynamic tissue which undergoes constant remodeling throughout the life span. Bone turnover is a measurement of bone tissue dynamics – such as the rate of mineral/matrix interchange and recuperation.[33]

You'll often find K2 included in bone formulas with vitamin D and calcium, given their synergistic effect on general bone health. Additionally, Cindy incorporated stretching techniques employed by a supportive physiotherapist, intake of a nervine herbal tonic, supplementation of a few other key minerals and age-appropriate stress management techniques. Her condition gradually became more bearable and less disruptive of her sleep. The initial prescription was no longer needed, and class performance significantly improved. Cindy continued being co-managed with the physiotherapist and a family therapist, which no doubt helped speed this positive turnaround.

I was glad that Cindy's grandma had looked beyond their initial situation for another opinion. Cindy has since continued growing minus agitating discomfort, and was able to resume her beloved gymnastics classes. This child wasn't making up stories about a phantom illness. It was fortunate that she stuck with her own intuition, to find the support she needed between family and health providers. Sometimes it takes a village approach and that's what was achieved in this case.

6.

Sickness And Society

*T*here is an argument that society needs illness as an anthropological matter. The theory is that illness is a result of societal and personal scripting; the role that illness plays varies within different cultures, among different individuals, within historical, geographical, genetic and social contexts.

In this light, does illness offer a means of judgement and personal identity? For instance, you might be more inclined to tell others you're suffering from diabetic complications than a sexually transmitted disease. People may think more sympathetically of you when suffering from period pain than the impact of obesity. Social pressures tend to condone certain conditions while rejecting others.

Despite great advances in the mental health arena, mental disorders can be subject to negative judgements and stigmatisation. Social exclusion and prejudice have long been prevalent because many people fear and misunderstand mental illness.

Wulf Rössler published a paper on this topic:

> For millennia, society did not treat persons suffering from depression, autism, schizophrenia and other mental illnesses much better than slaves or criminals: they were imprisoned, tortured or killed. During the Middle Ages, mental illness was regarded as a punishment from God: sufferers were thought to be possessed by the devil and were burned at the stake, or thrown in penitentiaries and madhouses where they were chained to the walls or their beds. During the Enlightenment, the mentally ill were finally freed from their chains and institutions were established to help sufferers of mental illness. However, discrimination reached an unfortunate peak during the Nazi reign in Germany when hundreds of thousands of mentally ill people were murdered or sterilised.[34]

Thankfully, humanitarian conditions have changed dramatically, to the extent that even public figures are willing to openly admit when they're struggling with anxiety, bipolar depression or the nuances of being on the autism spectrum.

Do you look at people differently if they're suffering certain ailments?

For example, would you look kindly upon an addict who had lost him or herself in their habit? Would you view their addiction as something out of their control? A genetic imposition, not their fault?

What if that person had grown up in an addictive family – be it addiction to illicit substances, toxic relationships, violent movies, cigarettes, or simply addiction to chocolate or one's smart phone?

In our world, we usually regard addicts as bad and self-indulgent people. Often they hurt their families, or let people down because their addiction has become the priority for them. It has to come first, because it's controlling them. I was once robbed of my entire paycheque and a few household goods by acquaintances I later discovered were heroin addicts, and through my work I've seen how terribly hard it is for an addict to stay clean. It isn't a pretty sight and evokes emotion and criticism, particularly if we cannot comprehend the psychology of addiction.

In an extract called 'Genes matter in addiction', Nora Volkow, MD, director of the National Institute on Drug Abuse stated: 'Understanding the complex interactions between the factors involved in drug abuse and addiction is critical to effective prevention and treatment.' With new data unfolding, physicians might soon be able to incorporate genetic tests in their practice, allowing them to better match specific treatments to individuals.

For example, Volkow explained that a certain type of dopamine receptor, known as D2, might someday be used to predict whether someone will become addicted to alcohol or cocaine. Brain imaging suggests that people with fewer D2 receptors are more likely to become addicted – and the number people have is, in part, genetically determined.

Of course, environmental factors also play a role. Volkow added, 'First, a person has to experiment with drugs, then he or she has to use them repeatedly. At that point, genetic vulnerability helps determine who winds up addicted'.[35]

From an outside perspective, it's easy to believe that an addict should simply control themselves and stop the vicious cycle of drinking to excess or using drugs – then there wouldn't be a problem. And yet it's proposed that 'at least half of a person's susceptibility to drug addiction can be linked to genetic factors'.[36]

This isn't to say that this category of individuals can't enjoy recovery and rehabilitation, but it will take ongoing mindfulness, self-control, community support and a bigger reason than the addiction to live for. That's a lot of variables, which may be difficult to line up.

There are endless high-functioning alcoholics and drug users in our society who wouldn't typically be identified as having a problem. For the most part, this is because they've become adept at keeping up appearances and hiding their secret. Walk into any drug and alcohol rehabilitation centre and you'll see many high achievers who've pushed through imbalance and overdrive sustained by 'crutches' of various sorts – the successful doctor addicted to codeine to function, the advertising executive with a cocaine habit or the mum volunteering at school tuck-shop, who endures her personal episodes of mental breakdown by hiding a flask of whisky in her handbag, secretly drinking day and night to cope.

If you've spoken to these people and realised how excessive and all-encompassing their reliance on drinking has become, you would wonder how they get through the day. Truth is, most don't. They make a mess of their lives, ruin kinships, have car accidents and destroy things for themselves and their loved ones. This is not a judgement, but a fact; it can become very hard to maintain such secrecy and drunkenness when others are relying on you to function sober. Likewise, for the people close to them it can feel very hard to continue giving unconditional love to those who are drowning in their addiction, because they either refuse or waste any well-meaning support given. Hence, their loved ones may turn them away; they then go deeper into their burrow of addiction, seemingly proving to others how hopeless they are.

Invariably, things unravel further and the addict crashes. Doing so can be the crisis that saves them, because they've hit bottom barrel, possibly lost everything (money, drivers licence, finances, marriage, friendships, job), and the only way up is via sobriety. Securing access to resources to help them with their disease is paramount.

Like with any other illness, slow and steady recovery is better than any attempt of a quick fix. In my clinic, I tell clients that for every year they have experienced a condition, they can expect a month to fully repair. So, if you've been suffering asthma for ten years, theoretically it could take up to ten months to restore your lungs and your total health to be asthma-free.

This slow burn is why most of us turn to a quick fix, shoot the messenger and soldier on. But when something is ruining or affecting our life, those months and the effort of letting our disturbances disturb us can be worth their weight in gold, because we're less likely to return to the place we came from and more likely to actively stop the 'two steps forward, one step back' pattern we've been stuck in. By sitting with our 'broken bits' and working to resolve them, we're more likely to enjoy lasting resolution – and not only that, but also an improved sense of self-empowerment, strength and resolve.

Drug and alcohol rehabilitation

When Doug first arrived in my clinic, he was using recreational drugs and drinking significant amounts of alcohol on a daily basis. His cheeks were ruddy and the sweat on his brow was evident.

Doug was anxious; straight vodka helped take the edge off his nerves. During our first session, I learnt that he wanted to wean off these habits but struggled to stop.

Doug is an ex-policeman. In his own words, he wished for a 'conflict-free world' where people could enjoy the safety of peace. Doug's work in law enforcement represented his belief in justice and fairness, of protecting the innocent; however, the cumulative effect of workplace trauma was wearing him down. Doug didn't need to share with me his horrible stories of sadness, violence and injustice. He sat on the edge of his chair fidgeting, explaining to me how he'd long struggled to sleep, and woke up with night sweats.

Without intending to, Doug found himself turning to drugs and alcohol as a means of emotional escape. He'd enjoyed periods of being focused on his fitness, but the alcoholic beverages and partying for temporary escapism always managed to creep back in. There were a few small health crises along the way, including liver problems, and his body was protesting louder and more frequently than ever before.

Incidentally, not long before Doug's first consultation, I'd begun working a little more frequently with addiction, so I was looking for fresh insights and perspectives on the topic, wanting to be best placed in supporting people like him in what can be their worst personal 'hour'.

I discovered other less traditional views abound, which take the onus away from the addict, and recognise the deeper metaphysical and emotional aspects at play. I learnt that addiction exists when we experience an inability to think of anything beyond what we're feeling. When our body is trying to experience something, and these feelings take over our thinking, addiction unfolds.

How does this occur? Our cells send imagery to the frontal lobe of our brain that tries to get us to eat the cake or smoke the cigar. Why? Because we're addicted to the biochemical reaction that occurs when we take that first bite, or inhale that smoke. This is when the hypothalamus excretes a certain chemical into the cells that allows us to feel a certain way (e.g. relaxed). And later, when our cells are starved of that compound, they send imagery to trigger us into wanting a repeat of that experience.

An addict naturally thinks the cake or cigar will fix their feelings. And the intellect is unable to override the emotions that may argue against this, given the force of the chemical wiring that pulls the addict back toward the experience. This 'hit' is temporary though, so it's important to try to fill that longing and urge with more sustainable options.

With Doug, it wasn't that he'd hit rock bottom or destroyed his life; the motivating factor for change was that he felt he was losing himself.

Whether it's an addiction or a temporary habit that's begun to take centre stage in our life, when we desire freedom from this pattern, the common thread is that we've identified the gap between who we know we can be vs who we've become. We're supposedly highly connected in modern society, but on the contrary – we commonly lack a sense of connection. The word 'disconnection' is raised, given we've identified the sense of losing ourselves in the process of our unhealthy habit. It's as if the addiction has taken over and is running the show.

Doug wanted peace in the world and inner peace for himself, but his life had begun to reflect the opposite reality. It was time to unravel that discord, so he decided to check into a drug and alcohol rehabilitation retreat and clinic. The journey of his sobriety didn't come without pain – although his family was ashamed of his predicament, Doug took the program seriously and continued with all the post-rehab necessities that were critical in avoiding relapse. With this came gradual increasing wellbeing. His body was repairing on the inside in ways that Doug previously thought were impossible. His liver was recovering, the acidity in his body reduced, his immunity strengthened, his eyes glowed, and his skin lost its yellow and flaccid appearance.

Doug had to both admit his own powerlessness to his addictions and believe in something bigger than himself for perspective and self-growth. This wasn't quick or easy to achieve and required connecting with mentors and other addicts who could relate with, monitor and support him.

Nowadays, Doug enjoys a new sense of self-satisfaction and belief that resonates more clearly with his greatest values. He's more the man he hoped to be. Nobody could have forced Doug to do the hard work involved in getting himself there. He had to make the choice himself and own his part in his downward spiral. His body had been telling him for a long time that enough was enough – presenting as poor digestion, insomnia, disruptive snoring, feeling on edge, and struggling with headaches and tremors. This meant he'd long been relying on a variety of pharmaceuticals to get through each day – anti-inflammatories, pain relief, sleeping pills, antacids and more. For a long time things weren't right, but his choice then was to ignore his moaning body, which showed him the lack of peace that existed in his life. Peace and justice were his highest values, so being able to obtain those feelings without compromising his sobriety was key.

Doug now exercises regularly and has become an early bird – a lifestyle change that's more conducive to his goals. He's involved in a Men's Shed in his local neighbourhood, bringing a sense of community and purpose beyond working life. Doug hasn't let his biology become his biography. He bravely accepts and manages the fact that he is an addict who needs to continue with self-insight measures, to avoid reverting to old ways of being.

Doug's story reminds us that if we lose our sense of self, even in a major and destructive way, it's never too late to rekindle a more validating hopeful connection with who we really want to be.

Health is wealth
– when one supplement achieves multiple outcomes

N-acetyl-cysteine (NAC)

NAC is a supplement that is widely used with a high safety profile. One of its best known actions is the contribution to glutathione production.[37] Glutathione is a primary antioxidant in our body and NAC is used to restore glutathione levels in cases of paracetamol overdoses and other pharmacologically induced glutathione deficiency states. When delivered intravenously or orally within 24 hours of overdose, NAC is effective at preventing liver toxicity.[38]

Glutathione sufficiency is critical to multiple diverse biological functions; NAC is used to reduce oxidative stress, particularly in cellular environments that are prone to oxygen damage. There's a great range of studies that have been undertaken on NAC's application in widely diverse health conditions; I could write a book on NAC alone. These include hepatic detoxification support (particularly if there is tissue damage), mitochondrial support (the part in cells that produces energy), and neurological support.

With mental health needs, NAC really shines[39] – studies cite NAC's efficacy in cases of ADHD, Alzheimer's, autism, mania, Parkinson's disease, traumatic brain injury, epilepsy, schizophrenia, bipolar disorder, behavioural concerns (such as drug addiction, nail biting and pathological gambling), obsessive-compulsive disorder (OCD), HIV infection,[40] noise-induced hearing loss and others.[41]

In respiratory health, given its mucolytic properties, NAC can reduce congestion and further support reproductive systems by helping to prevent miscarriage, with evidence on its efficacy with polycystic ovarian syndrome (PCOS).[42]

The ability of pathogens to become resistant to antibiotics is well reported, and in this realm NAC can be administered. This indicates possible benefits in the disruption of biofilms, which act to protect bacteria from antibiotics and other competing microbes – creating an environment within us that allows them to proliferate, unaffected by intervention.

NAC is an absolute mainstay in my dispensary and was successful for Doug and endless other clients who had detoxification and mental health needs as a high priority.

7.

The Kissing Disease That Lingers

I've always been driven to achieve goals and not rest on my laurels. Throughout childhood and my teen years, I had a real sense that any potential achievements were entirely my own responsibility; things wouldn't automatically be handed to me. Because I started school early, I was a year younger than my class peers. By the time I reached Year 12, it dawned on me that with this extra year below my belt, I could defer university for 12 months on completion of my High School Certificate, to work and build the funds I needed for my future career.

And work I did! Not only was I taking on the role of helping manage our household chores (as Mum had recently returned to a full-time position) I was cooking for us all (my mum, dad and sister) and looking after my horse.

I would finish a lunchtime waitressing shift at our local bistro, then go to the nearby shopping mall for my 5–9 pm retail role, then later in the week head off for a stint of modelling at a city nightclub (typically bikini or lingerie catwalks among the partying youngsters). I'd frequently submit articles to our local newspaper on topical events, volunteer at our community radio station (reading new stories or presenting the graveyard shift) and accept any acting roles I could (thanks to a supportive agent who knew how money-hungry university-aged kids like me were!).

The benefit of all this activity was a boosted sense of self-esteem and purpose. I was providing for myself and able to purchase my own first car.

After enjoying this feeling of being quite high on life, unfortunately I ended up hitting a low, suffering from a virus that didn't seem willing to dissipate. I'd been burning the candle at both ends, sustained by personal motivation despite my body becoming less keen to keep pushing on at such pace. Sometimes culling commitments is a positive and necessary exercise. I needed to start taking heed of this nagging virus, because it wasn't resolving under the status quo.

The saying 'I have glandular fever' could easily become a stamp for Year 12s who struggled to complete their end of secondary school exams. Like endless other adolescents, I too became a statistic for Epstein–Barr virus (EBV), more commonly known as glandular fever. This virus is spread via mucous exchange, so it's highly likely to be transmitted among teens through kissing.

Characterised by swollen glands, fever and profound fatigue, this state of stupor and discomfort may continue for months. For some unhappy sufferers, it can also develop into chronic fatigue syndrome (CFS), because it has not been fully resolved and the virus persists as a latent infection.

I've met many late teenagers who admit to having had glandular fever and would never wish to experience that again, as it can become so overwhelming that they never completely regain full energy and vitality – that is, unless the immune system is repaired and emotional factors of overwhelm are addressed.

In my case, I had to learn that it was okay to say no, given 'yes' was my default. I was working myself into the ground and my new boyfriend hardly saw me.

The label of busyness has become ingrained in our culture. Over-achieving, filling every spare gap of our days and weeks – juggling calendars, doing things quickly and getting frustrated when we're forced to *stop*.

It takes fortitude to switch this fast flow around for balance. To instil in our children the sense of equilibrium that nature brings to us: sunrise/sunset, winter vs summer, inhaling before exhaling, the tides that come in and go out. I see value in teaching our children the virtues of rhythm in our lives, such as daily or weekly rituals – whether it's pancakes every Sunday, or a shared family board game on Friday nights. Such small predictable gestures can bring us great benefits in feelings of grounding and belonging when our days are otherwise frantic. It's useful and health-inducing to stop leaning out and come back within, connecting or settling with family and community.

When my clients share with me how they struggle with panic attacks, I remind them of the tools I've learned: that the safest place to be is *in* our own bodies – and to try not to make what's happening to our bodies wrong, in our mind.

Breathing techniques shouldn't be overlooked for their perceived simplicity. A technique of breathing in for seven seconds and out for eleven seconds (my daughter likes to call it the 7/11 method) can remind us that if the world is going too quickly or seems a scary place, grounding ourselves within our bodies can bring stillness and perspective. At the very least, it offers a chance to regroup with yourself, for improved responses to your external circumstances. I've since discovered that the Buteyko method of breathing has literally transformed people's lives, resolving anxiety and asthma for endless Australians.

Accepting and embracing the art of not doing much seems unproductive and phlegmatic, but if the scales are always weighted to one side, the opposite extreme could be the perfect antidote. Glandular fever stopped me. I was forced to lay down and remain in a horizontal position because my muscles ached so much, it seemed they couldn't hold me upright. My lymph glands were swollen and sore. I was too exhausted to eat properly, frustrated with myself over doing so little, experiencing a fear of missing out yet having nothing left in the tank to change my circumstances

It was time to ask for help. I had to accept my vulnerability and turn to loved ones for support. This was also a chance for my parents to see that I needed to be carefully guided with my choices, even though I believed I was already an adult who could look after herself. Sometimes illness has a message for the whole family.

My little sister had to step up more in the household tasks, to help Mum and fill the gaps from me being unable to do anything. Dad had to support Mum and create more regulation in his own workload too. I didn't notice this all happening at the time but it's apparent now. My habits and resultant condition were symptomatic of our whole family dynamic. There were lessons for all of us in my state of sickness.

Illness for strength

Dethlefsen offers us fuel for thought to this end.

> Time was once when all parents knew that when a child survives a children's illness (all children's illness were infectious illnesses) it takes a step forward in development or maturity. After the illness the child is no longer the same as before. The illness has brought about a change that has made it more mature. But then it is not only childhood illness that have such a maturing effect. Just as the body itself emerges strengthened from each infectious illness that it survives, so the whole human being comes out of each conflict with greater maturity. For it is only challenges that make us strong and fit. All the world's highest cultures arose as a result of the severest challenges ... [43]

Viral shutdown

One of my clients, the gorgeous fair-skinned Mylee, had struggled with glandular fever for most of her last year at secondary school. This impacted her ability to attend social functions and sustain friendships. Mylee missed out on the graduation ball and her grades were so low that even the help of a tutor at home didn't save her from failing the year. Her mother joined her for many health-related appointments and was so invested in her daughter's return to normal function and health, that she slowly but surely became significantly drained herself.

A turning point after many months of mutual downs was when Mylee agreed to go interstate to stay with family friends, in a warmer and quieter environment and climate. This created a whole new level of worry for the loving mum, whose own life had become enmeshed with Mylee's needs.

Thankfully, they all adjusted to Mylee's absence and sure enough, the change of daily routine and sense of distance from perceived failures at school boosted Mylee's spirit enough that she was gaining strength and getting closer to recovery. It doesn't sound like a lot, but for a person who had never flown interstate, never left the family home and had been previously immersed in extracurricular actives and the rigours of her school routine, a trip away was a major shake-up. I believe having the courage to leave her parents and give them a chance to recuperate was quite courageous and insightful. This is not to suggest healing is simply a matter of taking a holiday; most of us know that problems usually follow if we try to run away from them.

Again, this case demonstrates how our wellbeing (or lack of it) not only changes our lives, but that of those around us. Mylee's mum had admitted to me later how she felt guilty about her lack of time for Mylee's younger sister, given her previous all-consuming focus on Mylee's needs. With her oldest offspring away, she could rectify that, helping to restore her own needs too. She's since become one of my clients too, now able to give herself that time, free from the role of Mylee's caregiver.

Another client, Juanita, in her 40s, still experiences flare-ups of her EBV, decades after it first presented. For her, this can present as fibromyalgia, exhaustion, swollen glands and ear infections. Treatment each time can require different methods, as her body changes and the virus presents in new ways. Although Chinese medicine or acupuncture may have helped Juanita years before, like I say to my clients, 'finding different pathways to the bottom of the rainbow' is the best road to recovery, at each recurrence. The body never stops feeding us signals of new imbalance and needs – being open, receptive and adjusting to these is recommended.

8.

Peak Performers And Injury

Sometimes our body stops us in different ways. These 'blows' can come out of seemingly nowhere and be very hard to grapple with – especially when competing at an elite level, eating well, consciously exercising, and literally depending on your body for career and self-purpose.

When self-identity is based around sporting success, injury can really shatter self-esteem. When a professional athlete experiences a physical setback, it may incite an emotional crash seemingly beyond the scope of the actual injury itself. The media frequently report on such stories where our pinnacle sportsmen and women appear to fall from grace. What are the lessons offered then? The gems of wisdom taught?

As a horse-rider myself, one who competed successfully at Pony Club and open levels for showing and eventing around my state, I know well the highs and lows of competition. I also understand the labour, organisation, endurance and flexibility called upon – not to mention the investment of money and time that goes into simply qualifying and getting to a horse-riding event. To some extent, certain things are out of your control too – like the weather, or the fact your horse is having a bad day. This tests even the most resilient and robust competitors.

$$*$$

Our beliefs impact our recovery

At the age of fourteen, Katherine Stewart (her true identity) was ranked 14th in the world as a show-jumper. This young Australian equestrienne could rise to the trot from the age of just two years old; perhaps an inevitable gift when born to a veterinarian father and a mum who is herself a very successful eventing rider.

Horses and other animals were always a big part of Katherine's life – riding, competing and selling them for business. While her dad always wanted her to have a back-up plan in terms of a future career, she didn't like that idea. Riding was the absolute focus, with all that came with those demands.

However, at age 17, feeling invincible after many hard-earned accomplishments, Katherine experienced a bad fall off a young horse, landing awkwardly on her back. Despite being rushed to hospital for x-rays, nothing was found to be broken at the time. Weeks later, she hadn't gotten any better, and there was a question over three possible fractures in her sacroiliac joint (pelvis) due to ligamentous damage.

Although falling off is a common risk to contend with, this set Katherine back in big a way; she says it was a 'shock to my system'. Katherine's mum recalls that she knew Katherine was struggling because she stopped singing in their family home. All of a sudden, there was no music that resembled Katherine's joyful spirit.

The incident had happened in May of that year, and after a few months of cortisone injections to help the repair process, in September of the same year she demonstrated her impressive determination and returned to riding. By October, Katherine qualified and went to the nationals, proudly representing our country.

In December of the same year, Katherine experienced another fall. This time it was much more significant – shattering the talus bone of her right ankle. This injury put her out of riding for over twelve months, and by her own admittance, 'the way I handled it was not good'.

In 'Coping With Injury: How High-Performance Athletes Mitigate the Biopsychosocial Consequences of Sports Injury', Kenny Chidozie Anunike, says:

> … injury becomes a major stressor in the athletes' life that dominates their thoughts, emotions, and actions. An injured athlete's rehabilitation process can be physically and mentally stressful. Physically, an athlete must adhere to rehabilitation set forth by a trained professional, properly re-train the muscles which have atrophied due to non-use, and consistently weight train the surgically repaired ligament or muscles far after the rehabilitation period has come to pass. But more importantly, the athlete's cognitive cycles must remain as optimistic as humanly possible to maintain the driving force behind his/her behaviours.[44]

Looking back now, Katherine can identify how these setbacks were a turning point for her – life was over, in terms of her riding career, which meant the young woman she had proudly become was no more. Her mind began spinning out of control with fear and worry – she felt like a hamster on a wheel, exhausted and getting nowhere.

Although she held onto her dream of competing in the global realm again, bigger and better, at that moment Katherine couldn't get out and be the best anymore – in fact, she couldn't even get out of bed. This was a huge shake-up for such a go-getting individual, enduring two months of isolation at home while shattered bones healed. At almost 18 during the school holidays/summer period, laying down with her leg elevated, of course it felt like the end of her world. It's understandable that Katherine experienced depression, anxiety and darkness during that time.

While recovering from the subsequent surgery, Katherine reviewed her eating habits, given she wasn't as active as usual. In her enforced idle position, she would read and absorb as much as she could about how to control her body and future, even from the bed.

With all that time on her hands, Katherine admits she became too self-focused – losing her identity as a rider, and the self-worth that naturally came with her competition-oriented lifestyle. The focus then became internal, to an unhealthy extent. She lost a great amount of weight, and although her new negative habits of over-analysing nutrients drained her energy, she was forced to look at what she was doing to herself.

Katherine realised she had to rebuild herself in many ways. Her drive was always to function at top level, but now the realisation had dawned on her that a more holistic approach to life was necessary.

It took a long time to develop a more balanced mindset and approach to her entire life, beyond the immediate future. After Katherine's ankle healed, she went to Europe to work with horses at a more sedate level than her typical pace. She was travelling and enjoying life, and participating with horses in a different way than her entire childhood journey had entailed.

Eventually returning home, Katherine threw herself into various, non-horse related jobs and gently explored other possibilities for herself, alongside her partner and beloved dog.

Katherine is now a well established motivational speaker, qualified occupational therapist, businesswoman and mentor for younger horse-riders. She is certain that her forced self-review and subsequent dabble into other different working environments – financial planning, transport and logistics, hospitality, agriculture and study – gave her valuable insights she wouldn't have otherwise gained while ploughing onward on the path of non-stop competition.

The horse-rider route was always her planned journey, and yet falling off that road gave her a new sense of integrity and clarity on a broader path. She learned to surround herself with motivated people, and discovered the great impact exercise and diet has on not only the body, but also the brain.

She now teaches her 'ten fundamentals to a sensational life', sharing how we can be responsible for our own thoughts to pave the kind of life we envision. Her experience with injury was the hardest part of her life by far. And yet, although it may sound clichéd, Katherine insists she also considers that experience of 'brokenness' as her best experience too.

It changed my path; I now am able to feel genuine gratitude for the challenges life continues to deliver – I now love to be a learner – I am truly grateful for that opportunity of learning too. So any speed hump or roadblock I come across allows me to embrace the challenge to be a more successful and happy person. I don't baulk at the hard times anymore, I accept them with open arms.[45]

Katherine's story is a striking one because she was clearly a driven individual from the outset. Like with many of us, having a sense of control over her body and future was always assumed. Without full health, her whole identity was at risk of falling apart. Having worked with a couple of Olympians and some iron-men/women, I've noticed a few standout features of people like Katherine. The first is their ability to push through discomfort, enabling them to achieve at such high levels, beyond what many others are able to accomplish. Mindset is a major basis to success.

Chidozie Anunike notes:

Athletes that excel at their sport often deal with pain on a regular basis, even when they are not injured. Because of this, it is common for them to try to return to their normal activities more quickly than they usually would following an injury, despite the pain that the injury is causing. This can lead to poor physical and psychological health outcomes for the athlete. (However) athletes have a higher tolerance for pain than normally active adults. Their ability to withstand pain (pain tolerance) is significantly greater. This is a notable distinction because it's not that athletes feel less pain, they are just able to deal with it better.[46]

Interestingly, pain in this case is not seen as an entirely physical stressor; it can be used as a motivator.

Another notable factor is that peak performers perhaps more quickly identify maladaptive ways of dealing with injury vs what is useful for them to bounce back. No doubt part of this is not only the pressure they put on themselves but also sheer necessity – if functioning physically is the source of your income. Chidozie Anunike again:

> It is not uncommon for people to go through denial when something devastating happens to them. This is the first of two primary maladaptive ways of dealing with injury. Denial is our brain's way of protecting us against extremely hurtful or disturbing situations. Someone going through denial tries to convince him or herself that what they have experienced is not real or that the consequences of the situation aren't as bad as they seem. While most professionals don't encourage people to stay in denial, it can sometimes be a helpful coping method. For example, it can help a terminally ill patient to maintain an optimistic outlook on prolonging his or her life.[47]

It's clear that in many cases, athletes will draw on this 'mind over matter' approach, harnessing their will to rise faster and stronger out of injury and illness.

In his book, *The Adversity Advantage: Turning Everyday Struggles Into Everyday Greatness*, Dr Stoltz clearly agrees, noting 'setbacks are inevitable, but misery is a choice'.[48] I would suggest that when someone overcomes a great personal health crisis, it's not always about luck but micromanagement and resolve as well – something all of us could draw upon if we find ourselves in a similar situation.

9.

Dietary Choices — Fueling Vs Starving

*I*t's a distinct privilege to be in a position to pick and choose what we eat, not only for basic nourishment but for aesthetic, ethical or personal beliefs. When I was a young recruit to the corporate world, one of the first things I did with my new income was to sponsor a child via World Vision. I enjoyed receiving photos of my sponsored South American girl, gaining perspective and gratitude for my comparatively salubrious life here, in a country where food and clean water is abundant, quality health services are readily accessible and opportunities for girls and women abound.

Now as a mother, I always try to offer my own children comparisons of what their meals might look like if they were in a less developed country or experiencing famine. Perspective is everything.

Despite best intentions and efforts, some clients I've met in my years of practice have unwittingly starved themselves of vital nutrients – despite, in some cases, being overfed. How can this happen?

Wearing a brightly coloured scarf and tie-dyed leggings, Ellen literally bounced into the clinic when I first met her; she was so full of enthusiasm and readiness for the session. Her main complaint was lethargy and iron deficiency, but you wouldn't have guessed it. She spoke confidently and loudly, bringing a basketful of supplements that she'd been taking. Ellen then pulled out her laptop and showed me a spreadsheet she'd compiled of her menstrual cycle and diaries of symptoms and food consumption – with graphs and charts demonstrating where, in her calculations, she could be missing certain nutrients.

Initially I was thrilled, imagining how this client would no doubt be very compliant and respond readily to treatment, given such focused attention and pre-prepared homework. And yet over time, we discovered certain gaps in Ellen's regimen, which were having a major detrimental impact on her wellbeing.

Anorexia and bulimia

Ellen had a history of eating disorders, and self-diagnosed OCD (obsessive-compulsive disorder). Her reflex to purge was instant and constant, even from the very thought of food passing her lips. I'd seen her do this with various liquid herbals we had sampled in clinic too. Ellen simply ran to the clinic toilet, wiped her face and returned without as much as a blink. It was apparent this was a process she'd learnt to manage without fuss.

To an extent, I could relate. During my teen years I was fond of the gym, carefully training 5–6 days weekly monitoring each food item that I consumed. I could tell you to the gram how much I weighed and what I could lift or carry with any given muscle group in my body when working out. After a rigorous ongoing schedule of fitness classes and endurance type activities, my body fat percentage had dropped to 5%. Given the standard body fat mass range for a healthy young female[49] is 19–22%, it's little wonder that my body could no longer menstruate; I didn't have enough fat to produce healthy female hormones for a proper cycle.

Despite my physical output, I recall avoiding dietary fat and counting calories and protein portions around the clock. My closest friends were also body-builders obsessed with their physique and nutrition, so this intense discipline was relatively simple for me to manage. We'd have three egg-white shakes, weigh our chicken breast fillets and broil our vegetables. It was a healthy and enjoyable pursuit, but such rigidity was erring on the unhealthy side (in my case at least).

While in hindsight I can see that I was trying to prove a sense of self-drive and control, and I was successful in my fitness goals, I now realise the extent to which current health norms play out and influence our choices. Back then, I was also modelling as a means to complement my casual income at various retail and hospitality jobs, before I began university. Those were the times when Elle McPherson ('The Body') was spread across media, so a frail, skinny model was certainly not the bankable body type. I was naturally strong and aspired to be athletic, like Elle. And yet at one of my 'go sees' where I shared my portfolio and was again asked to parade in bikinis before a panel of judges, the feedback to my agency was that I was too thin and to come back when I had gained a couple of kilos!

Anorexia nervosa is a serious illness that has a diverse range of effects on the body and mind. It carries the potential to become a severe psychological disorder and, unsurprisingly, is increasingly common among young women where cultural expectations encourage women to be thin. Fuelled by popular fixations with thin and lean bodies, anorexia also affects a growing number of men, particularly athletes and those in the military. A big part of the satisfaction mixed into this is the self-control, which is why people with obsessive personalities (excessive need to control their personal environment) tend to be affected by eating disorders. [50]

Anorexia is frequently associated with several other medical problems, ranging from infections and general poor health to life-threatening conditions. One of the most common effects is hormonal changes, impacting reproductive function and reducing estrogen levels (required for a healthy heart and bones). Thyroid function is altered and stress hormones are higher while growth hormones are reduced. Abnormalities in brain chemistry occur too. Changes in serotonin levels, the brain chemical that regulates appetite, may contribute to other symptoms such as depression, impulsiveness, obsessive behaviour, or related mood disorders.

If the person is purging (self-imposed vomiting and bulimia) this process may deplete tryptophan, an amino acid necessary for the creation of protein, vitamins and digestive enzymes – all crucial elements for a healthy body. Resultant symptoms include cold hands and/or feet, fatigue and fainting, increased dental decay, loss of periods/menstrual cycle, heart and kidney problems and fine hair appearing on the face and body.[51]

People with anorexia are terrified of becoming obese and refuse to maintain a normal weight, putting themselves in danger of starvation. While I would never have identified myself as having an eating disorder in my 'fitness freak' years, given I ate a great deal and was not purging, there were certain threads that I could relate to as I worked with Ellen.

To date, I have worked with over a dozen clients with a history of eating disorders. Sufferers actually see themselves as overweight even when they're so extremely thin that their bodies are becoming debilitated. 'Mind over matter' rings true here – there is a shutdown of what they are feeling physiologically, because their opposing thoughts are so determined and strong.

Ellen was no longer limiting her food intake. However, she experienced ongoing problems with mood imbalance and iron deficiency, to the extent that she often ended up at her doctor's for an iron infusion. There were times when she simply couldn't get her body out of bed, the fatigue was so extreme – impacting her ability to work and worrying her family. Ellen had opted for a vegan diet a few years earlier and she was certainly health-conscious, putting great effort into eating 'clean' organic foods.

We're fortunate now that there exists a great deal more awareness around veganism and vegetarianism. There is also an exorbitant variety and abundant availability of non-animal sourced quality foods to ensure you can meet all nutrient needs. Hemp seed oil is a complete protein and one of nature's richest source of amino acids. It's also rich in magnesium and zinc, plus omega-3 and -6 fatty acids, and is low-allergen and highly digestible. Chia seeds are relatively good in protein content, antioxidants and healthy fats too; they are so versatile for both savoury and sweet preparations.

While it's honourable to avoid animal cruelty and eat in a manner that resonates with one's personal philosophies, particularly given environmental factors of meat production, the body is a complex machine with endless mechanisms, so it takes commitment and awareness to sustain your health when cutting out major sources of protein and animal-derived omega-3 essential fats. Of course, it's possible to thrive as a vegan. I know ultra-marathon runners who are happily vegan; they manage to do this well and have incredible drive, organisation and commitment to living large.

As with Ellen, a few of my vegan clients are students who chose to cut out animal sources from their meals for mostly ethical reasons; however, perhaps they weren't prepared for any possible factors such as travel, where your usual food sources aren't as readily available and you end up missing core nutrients. Ellen had travelled most of South America, Mexico and later South Africa. My tip: don't make major health commitments if you're away from home and unable to achieve the vital necessities that change entails.

Infertility and endometriosis

A low-fat diet starves your nervous system of fuel for normal healthy activity. Essential fats are named thus for a reason; they're vital for cell function, including our neurotransmitters. That's why fish oil is usually prescribed by naturopaths and nutritionists for depression.

Incidentally, fish oil has also been shown to assist with fat loss (see articles on this topic on my website, http://julieseamer.com/fish-oil-for-fat-loss/), something I didn't know when I was younger, and has long been a key supplement in part of my weight loss programs in clinic since.

Tammy offers us another example of unexpected nutritional deficiency, despite being a health-conscious person. A client in her mid-thirties who came to see me a few years ago, she had long been on a healthy vegan and macrobiotic diet, maintained a high-intensity marketing position and was experiencing anxiety. Tammy was taking the oral contraceptive pill, and hoped to stop this prescription to conceive a baby.

At the time of her first visit, Tammy was fatigued both mentally and physically. Her immediate health goals were to manage and overcome debilitating menstrual pain, obtain regular menstrual cycles, then fall pregnant. However, in her own words Tammy's exhaustion and frayed nerves seemed to be blocking the flow to achieving these goals.

As part of my standard initial naturopathic consultation, I not only assess the medical history and constitutional tendencies, but look closely at nutritional status – what is being ingested, absorbed and utilised, discovering if anything is potentially lacking. Nutritional deficiency often plays a part in driving ill health. In Australia, one would assume we should all have nutrient-rich bodies, given our abundant food sources; I argue we're more likely to be over-fed yet commonly starved of vital nutrients. It doesn't take much to upset the balance if one key element is missing in your diet – particularly if this absent piece of the puzzle has lingered long-term, creating disrupted biochemistry. Equally, long-term pharmaceutical use can deplete our nutrient status; this is why supplementation is important as part of a complementary plan, and to safely optimise the benefits of your medication.

Despite going to great lengths to eat well, Tammy presented with significant nutritional deficiencies – possibly impacted by, among other things, decades of oral contraceptive pill use. The main nutrients depleted by this medication are vitamin A, the B vitamins and the trace mineral zinc. Essential fats were also lacking, something we became aware of when later discovering that Tammy had endometriosis. These adhesions on her uterus would potentially cause ongoing infertility (and further pain) unless addressed.

By working on restoring the underlying deficiencies, rebalancing her female hormones and reducing the inflammation beyond her endometrium, over several months the condition was subsiding. Gynaecology sessions were also part of this management plan, along with the suggestion to obtain subsidised access to a mental health therapist of her choice.

It takes commitment to overhaul your eating regimen, particularly when cultural, ethical and familial factors play a part in that lifestyle choice. Although Tammy had been previously avoiding sources of animal-derived foods, she was willing to alter that, if doing so meant that she could get closer to achieving her ultimate desire of falling pregnant. I mention this because, of her own accord, Tammy and her husband tried adjusting to a paleo-based diet for four weeks. This was almost a total turnaround of how they ate before as vegans.

And despite the effort of shopping at different places and pre-preparing meals for the working week, plus having to stay committed to this during corporate events and work lunches, the results spoke for themselves. At our next session together, Tammy happily reported that her energy had returned, clarity of mind was restoring, and a lust for life and libido was emerging – creating the ideal conditions for trying to conceive.

Some months later in a subsequent joint consultation, I was surprised and happy to learn that she and her husband had made a big life decision – to pack up their material items, leave their jobs and take a whole year off to travel around Australia. Tammy's intention was to remove herself from the source of stress at work and to stop intentionally focusing on ovulation cycles, which was making falling pregnant more of a chore than an incidental side effect of the couple's intimacy. They both wanted to 'live in the moment' and allow nature to take its course. They conceded that if it meant that a baby wasn't forthcoming, they were willing to accept and live with that outcome.

It was pleasing to receive postcards of their travel. Just before Christmas, on their return, Tammy re-booked with me, bringing wonderful news: they were expecting their first baby! I now witness happy pictures on social media of their growing family, a fortunate outcome thanks in part to some personal shifts and tough decisions they were both willing to embrace.

It's been useful to explore such cases, taking diagnostic comparisons of the impacts of vegan vs paleo diet, and how different meal plans impact key inflammatory markers, oxidative stress/ageing, metabolic syndrome, cholesterol, iron and vitamin B12 levels, gut integrity, body pH, etc. In other words, how food can be medicine, or the cause of discord, depending on the individual's needs at the time of implementation. While I don't advocate any particular elimination of an entire food group from your diet – or opting for a meat-based diet if being vegetarian/vegan suits you best – for this family it was about exploring what being 'healthy' meant to them. I don't know if they've returned to veganism.

Whatever the situation, as I always say to my clients, 'It's your health, your choice.' (Although, please, be informed and brutally honest with yourself about the choices you make!)

My wise yoga teacher often repeats the following mantra: 'I surrender control. I submit to the natural flow.'

There certainly is power in this state of being, if we can manage to let go of being in the driver's seat a while. I would wager that most of the time, many of us are fighting against ourselves, our circumstances, the traffic, our slow wi-fi service, the annoying people at the grocery checkout line, the irritating small niggling pain in our neck that we haven't got time to resolve, and so on. Sometimes, going against the flow wastes energy and resolve.

What if you truly listened to and surrendered to whatever your ailments are calling you to?

10.

Oncology Care

Sometimes in life, you come across a kindred spirit, and feel instantly close to and understood by one another, despite having only met. Emma was one of those friends for me.

We shared a love for horses, a connection with the community and lands of the green wedge of Melbourne, and a desire to make a difference for others faced with major health hurdles.

Devoting many years of service to her nursing career, Emma worked with people who suffered spinal injury – helping them to live beyond the confines of their body's current physical state. In this pursuit, she witnessed miracles daily – whether that was someone overcoming paralysis or being able to move a certain body part, intentionally, after extreme injury and pronounced immobility.

Emma coined the phrase 'Health on Purpose'. In her experience, if we have a purpose to be healthy – if we intend to move beyond our perceived or actual limitations – there can be no looking back.

That is, our health and lives would be purposeful. She loved to start conversations about the transformative effect disease and illness can have on us, and this sparked a fire within her patients for their hopeful recovery.

Emma was inspired by Dr Joe Dispenza, the chiropractor from the US who overcame major spinal injury himself and has since become a best-selling author and world leader in self-development circles. Emma introduced me to his remarkable personal story of post-paralysis renewal, plus his passion to explore and uncover the paradigm of mind and body. Emma had attended many of Dr Joe's lectures around the globe, became his master coach for Australia and employed these lessons into her vocation at a rehabilitation hospital for those living with the effects of brain and spinal injury. Emma authored her own book too: *Diagnosis to Recovery: The Path to Wholeness*.

I believe Emma's case is important to share because she personally encountered lung cancer, while supporting her mother who also had lung cancer before Emma was diagnosed. Emma was a non-smoker, so her diagnosis came as an unwelcome shock – particularly at a time when her energies were directed to supporting her mum, who was undergoing chemotherapy. In her own words, 'There's nothing like being told you're going to die to make you finally live.'

From my experience, cancer is indiscriminate – some people manage to stay in remission while others, despite their best efforts and whole-hearted attempts to overcome the ravaging effects of the disease, sadly do not 'beat it'. As is likely for most people nowadays, I've been touched by cancer more than desirable. I work within oncology occasionally, drawing on evidence-based nutritional supplements that have been proven to safely enhance the cytotoxicity and effectiveness of chemotherapy, yet markedly reduce the side effects for those undergoing treatment.

Statistics show the high percentage of people who seek out complementary medicines when dealing with cancer.[52] Whatever regimen my clients choose, I ensure that everything is shared with their oncologist and that a green light is given before proceeding. As always, it's about shared care, striving for the best outcomes in a safe and measured manner.

In Emma's words:

> What doesn't help is to ignore the emotional and mental impact of disease by treating your physical symptoms alone. On the other side of illness there is always wholeness.

> There are differences between treating, curing and healing. Treating is relieving a symptom, curing is overcoming the disease and healing encompasses the whole person.[53]

Typically, a few of my clients are actively having chemo or radiotherapy; many others are on the other side of that, attending return consultations to maintain their wellbeing beyond their initial cancer diagnosis.

Emma chose me to be one of her health practitioners when her first diagnosis came about. From the outset, she had the mindset of a winner, commenting 'disease and pain asks you to look inside yourself'.[54]

She set out to review what was most precious in her life, carefully decluttering and protecting herself from outside noise/influence that wasn't supportive of her healing process.

Later in her book, she wrote:

> The greatest of treatments simply cannot work as
> effectively when they are up against the body's innate
> stress response, which takes over and continues to cause
> breakdowns ... So what are the 'best' conditions for
> your body to heal? It needs a break from whatever was
> constantly occurring which triggered this damage in the
> first place. It sounds logical, right? Most people change
> diets, stop smoking or get more rest but the one vital
> element that often gets bypassed in chronic disease is to
> change your inner world.[55]

Emma determined that meditation would become part of her daily
rhythm, to cope with the endless tests and the stress of being on
the other side of the hospital bed, and as a means to manage her
own fears and overwhelm. She strongly felt that by stilling her mind
and controlling the only thing she could – her thoughts – that she'd
be better equipped to deal with the daily rigours of chemotherapy.

> Disease is your initiation into personal leadership ...
> Although it feels like your world is falling apart, this is
> precisely where the hero inside us has space to emerge.[56]

Evidently, Emma was drawing on her own inner reserves in an
attempt to push through her gruelling schedule of treatments.
She used some of that time to make note of her personal cancer
journey, which later become her book.

Remarkably, Emma enjoyed remission from lung cancer within a
year. She was outstanding in the coups she achieved. At one point
there was threat of having to endure a blood transfusion, but

after vigilantly taking a blood-building liquid herbal I'd prepared, doing everything her oncologist suggested and working around the clock to focus on being as positive she could be, sure enough, her blood results came back healthier and she dodged that bullet. This allowed her to travel overseas with her partner and continue seeking answers to her own questions on recovery.

In subsequent months, we were scheduled to meet as she wasn't feeling too well; however, Emma didn't arrive for the appointment. She didn't answer my messages, which was out of character and concerned me. The next day I learnt that she'd had a stroke; the tumours had gone to Emma's brain, causing some brain damage. This was a wretched blow and I was greatly worried about her prognosis.

Over the next two months, Emma was in palliative care in our nearby oncology-specialising hospital and, once again, she impressed me with her spunk. Despite being dosed with morphine and unable to move part of her body, Emma still worked on achieving the impossible, wiggling her toes for me during a visit, giggling and impressed at herself.

She had moments of being very lucid and would send me the most determined SMS messages, despite having to stay hospitalised over the entire Christmas and summer period. I knew from experience that even looking at a mobile phone screen can be difficult due to the effects of chemotherapy and other procedures. But she still managed to communicate with the outside world and her network of friends, including me. In my view, Emma's fortitude and trust in her body was nothing short of phenomenal.

I'm a glass half-full kind of person, but I'm also realistic about how deadly cancer can be.

In Emma's case, while I knew she was in the best hands – and as a nurse herself, she was always acknowledging the teams of staff around her – I worried about her future. Among her immediate community, we aimed to raise funds so she could go home and rest in peace, should that possibility be available to Emma. The donations were used to renovate her house and bathroom to allow wheelchair access. Over the next month, Emma literally willed herself to enjoy small incremental improvements – in being able to hold solid food down, in being able to talk more readily, in being able to move more body parts. She just didn't give up.

> Catastrophic experiences ... show us that there are qualities within ourselves that have the power to sustain us through seemingly impossible situations.[57]

> Our inner resources are just as powerful as the physical treatments (such as chemo) to get well.[58]

Within weeks, I received some great news from Emma – she was being transferred to her place of work, the rehabilitation hospital, for physiotherapy and exercises to ready herself in going home. This was remarkable and very exciting. I tried a few times to visit, but her rehabilitation schedule was so full it was near impossible to fit me in!

Again, I quietly wondered: in her shoes, could I be so impassioned and eager to prove everyone wrong and continue to get better, when any hopeful expectations of my improvement were lacking? Emma wasn't willing to allow her quality of life to change. Even while crippled in her ailing body, her trust in wholeness was evident.

A little while after this, Emma's partner called, saying she'd developed a nasty chest infection and the news was that if she didn't improve within 24 hours it was back to palliative care, not home. At her request and with his personal permission, I immediately prepared a bundle of safe and powerful supplements to take to her. As my son wasn't well, I couldn't go into the hospital and see Emma when I arrived, so her friend came out to collect the items. At this point, I was struggling to hide my concern; it seemed that every time Emma rose above her circumstances, something else would challenge any hard-earned progress.

Emma's friend Doug, who was with her during that time, is also a spiritual person, a soul with a calming energy. He assured me that I could trust Emma's journey, and that by surrendering to her reality would be in keeping with her approach – she had no resistance, only trust in her body and what it was telling her.

At that moment I recalled something she'd said to me earlier in her cancer journey: 'It's not my job to cure my broken body, Jules … my job is to get out of the way so it can do what it's designed to'.

Reading her words now reinforce these sentiments:

> The body shows us what happens in the mind and knows how to correct the imbalance the minute we let go of resisting our old ways. It is normal to resist something that we think will bring us suffering. Resisting the experience of disease was effectively keeping myself trapped in the fear, anger and frustration that I came to see were underlying my cancer.[59]

> Surrender doesn't mean to be inactive in your recovery ... to surrender is to let go, not give up.[60]

> When we take our focus from the experience at hand and deliberately look for what we are grateful for, we release hormones of repair and restoration. From a calm, grateful state of mind, the nervous system relaxes, the body's self healing mechanisms are turned on and healing is possible.[61]

> The very energy of 'fighting' your illness or the situation you're in actually contributes to making you sick ... It seems counter intuitive to accept things we don't want but fighting it doesn't work either. It makes things worse. For example 'a war' on cancer infers something is wrong and sends your body that message.[62]

Admittedly, while I was moved by her sentiments, this also rattled me. I was indignant on behalf of her – I wanted to battle the disease, to prevent it from annihilating my friend. My reaction was defensive, fear-based and not accepting of Emma's reality. Even with calm, grounded Doug before me, part of me wanted to cry.

I felt smashed by the unexpectedness of this nasty disease that was impacting my friend – robbing her of time spent with loved ones. I wished for her to be better and I didn't want her to suffer with sickness anymore. I longed to see Emma back in her home among the gum trees, not in these sterile hospital spaces.

I felt sad but also knew that she wouldn't want me to be, so I tried to change my perspective and stop panicking. Taking these musings home with me, it was another sense of relief when Emma messaged

24 hours later that she was feeling considerably better and able to go home the next day. I couldn't quite believe it. How impressive! I'd dreaded the worst of news, so this was perfect. Going home would be the ideal recovery environment for my friend and her inner circle, who were supporting her around the clock. We agreed to share a celebratory cuppa soon, and I continued to muse about Emma's journey as the next week unfolded.

Two weeks went by and I hadn't heard from Emma or her partner. I was comforted knowing that she was home and no doubt fuelled by the serenity there. Then, the news arrived. Emma transitioned from her body on the subsequent weekend, a sun-dappled Sunday afternoon, hand in hand with her partner and best friend, in the comfort of her own house.

This news was devastating. In my mind Emma was a leader, wise beyond her years. She knew in her very essence that we're all masters of our own destiny. It didn't seem right that she should be taken away from us like this, although I knew I had to surrender – as she was always teaching me to.

Like with any loss of a loved one, Emma's passing reiterated the sobering reality of our human mortality, from which none of us can escape. I wanted my friend to stay here forever, as the mighty survivor she always managed to be. I ruminated and cried for a long while. If anyone could beat an awful disease, Emma of all people could.

Though, who is to say that Emma wouldn't have enjoyed her unexpected remission, had she not been so prepared to tune in to what her body and mind needed? Perhaps she wouldn't have had the peace of dying at home and never enjoyed the extra little blessings she created for herself, given her attitude and efforts in learning from her illness?

Knowing Emma, I have no doubt that she was still accessing her subconscious – choosing how to respond to her condition, not letting it to take control of her, and instead allowing and trusting.

It hit me too that unconditional love of oneself means to love our life, our bodies, our ugly symptoms, the pain and hardships – even during or especially when inflicted by a nasty condition. Kindly. Unconditionally.

No matter the fact she'd spent days, weeks and months within hospital walls, nights in beds that weren't her own – she still managed to marvel at the little blessings. Emma chose to have gratitude when could wriggle a finger, move her toes, stomach food or hold her head up to drink. There was always a little joke too. Laughter is healing. Thankfulness is love in action. All the way through, Emma was loving her life, her body, her situation.

> We are wired to approach life with a linear formula that results in our problems being solved in a certain amount of time. For example, if you have a headache (problem), then you take a tablet (solution) which will give you relief (result).[63]

> The reality of cause-and-effect is what we have been taught. However, in more complex situations such as chronic illness, this approach doesn't always work due to the increased complexities of the situation. We are multi dimensional creatures. Chronic illness is not a linear experience and so, it requires us to open up to the wider issues'. 'The mindset of 'thinking yourself to a greater reality' is never more relevant than when your

life is threatened. It's not to just support you through an experience like this, but to also determine the physical outcomes you experience.[64]

Only a month before Emma's passing, we also lost my late partner's sister Kristy to stage four cancer. This too felt like a great injustice, given she was such a beacon of light, who lived by honourable principles and led a healthy existence. Throughout her years of tackling the disease, often in gruesome circumstances given the nastiness of stage 4 presentations, Kristy never let us cry for her; she was doggedly optimistic and refused to see anything but the bright side of life. Even when they were draining litres of horrid fluid out of her swollen organs as the cancer spread, she would find a way to make a joke about it all, and continually thank her lucky stars for all the small blessings she could find in her life. It surely takes a special kind of person to be so brave, bright and selfless.

I'd known Kristy since our Pony Club days in Seville, Victoria – precious memories. She passed away the same age as her brother had, six years after him, only a few days before his anniversary. That cancer eventually took her from us has been a cruel hardship to endure, because she was extremely close to Scott, and so had already been through heartache in losing her sibling to mental illness. Now, she was leaving behind three gorgeous children and her devoted husband, who is the kindest man – leaving a hole that can never be filled, for him or any of us who knew and loved Kristy, especially her parents. Heartbroken is an understatement of how I felt about this.

Life can be unfair. We can embrace it with both hands and still be dealt cards that aren't to our liking, as Emma and Kristy were forced to accept. Maybe their spirits grew too large for their mortal bodies? In both cases, their individual responses to disease taught me things I may never have learnt otherwise. At the very least, I'm deeply humbled and thankful. Their lives have had a life-changing impact on those of us who carry their memories dear to our hearts.

11.

When Our Bodily Dysfunctions Become Unmanageable

*O*riginally developed in Sweden, phenomenography studies the variations in ways that people look upon, experience, or understand phenomena in the world around them. In other words, an experience, while simultaneously objective and subjective, is as much an aspect of the object as it is of the subject.[65]

Research in this area aimed to identify the different ways chronic illness can be experienced by patients. The findings found that patients' experiences of chronic illness can be described in terms of a different lived body, a struggle with identity and self-esteem, a diminished lifeworld, and a challenging reality.[66]

Illness and overwhelm

As a natural health practitioner, I've always been motivated to 'walk my talk'. Thankfully, my late fiancé-to-be was health-conscious and interested in nutrition too.

Scott was a childhood friend who had similarly become a parent and unfortunately divorced in later years, as I had. We reunited as pals after a chance meeting when I was thirty-nine. Over the following months, we supported each other in the various trials and emotional heartaches involved with co-parenting as a divorcee.

Scott's girls were in the later years of primary school. His younger daughter had leukaemia from infancy, although thankfully enjoyed a full recovery by ten years of age. Hence, wellness was a big focus for him and long had been. He also managed his own food sensitivities with a gluten-free and lactose-free diet. Protein smoothies, salads, eggs and vegetable stir-fries were among his favourite fuel. As a secondary school physical education teacher, hiker and surf life saver with a busy lifestyle, fitness was important and an absolute priority. Still, I learnt through Scott how debilitating seemingly small nagging health complaints can become, even if you're physically robust.

Scott endured back pain daily. The spaces between his vertebrae were compounding and before a hiking trip to do the famous Kokoda track, he had to receive an injection of cortisone to keep functioning.

At home, it wasn't only the chronic pain affecting him. Managing food sensitivity may not sound debilitating but when you're unable to pinpoint exactly what your body is reacting to, and then find yourself unable to sleep most nights, crippled in digestive pain – the days afterward surely feel long and hard. We noticed that if we ate at restaurants and there was a chance of MSG food flavourings or other artificial preservatives in a meal, Scott's stomach would bloat to monstrous proportions and the subsequent discomfort and disruptions to his life would have a ripple effect on everything, impacting his ability to cope with day-to-day stress.

We lose more of our precious dads, brothers, sons, uncles and nephews to suicide than disease. Sadly, I was soon to become familiar with the devastating after-effects of this statistic when my partner ended his life. This happened when I was mid-way through pregnancy, carrying our son, Liam. It perplexed me that we went from sharing an enjoyable meal together one night, watching a funny movie on TV, then waking early for an invigorating walk, hand in hand, discussing the problems of the world – to never seeing each other again. Life went from normal to a living nightmare within a matter of hours.

As the one left behind, the what-ifs, regrets, sadness and pain of loss are sometimes all too much to comprehend. But one thing has become clear to me from this experience: health problems shouldn't be ignored. With Scott, all the little complaints were stacking up so much that they became a load too heavy to bear – and nothing was enough to help tip the scales in Scott's favour. Medication alone couldn't switch his wiring enough to offer the fast results he needed. So, when clients are sitting in my treatment room and sharing the fact they feel unable to cope or are at the end of their tether, I listen willingly and feel gratitude for the chance to address their whole state of health – mental, spiritual and physical. It may just be the necessary conversation to save them from sinking into despair.

As a community of human beings, we needn't shy away from reaching out to others with care. The now famous survivor of his own suicide attempt, Kevin Hines, became a renowned advocate for such hope, sharing this message to the world with his documentary *Suicide: the Ripple Effect* and memoir *Cracked, Not Broken: Surviving and Thriving after a Suicide Attempt.*

As thousands of others have sadly done, Hines jumped off the Golden Gate Bridge in San Francisco in September 2000. At the time, he'd been suffering from bipolar depression and was hearing voices in his head, telling him he was worthless. During the bus trip to the bridge on the fateful day, Hines was wishing valiantly for just one person to reach out and ask if he was okay. Despite his wailing and pacing up and down across the bridge for 45 minutes, passing endless others, nobody acknowledged him or dared to ask if anything was the matter. This convinced him it was the right thing to do – and yet, despite his free-fall of around 73 metres in just four seconds, reaching 120 kilometres per hour on impact, he miraculously resurfaced from the water below. The moment his fingers left the railing, he felt instant regret. Despite crushing his spinal vertebrae and breaking an ankle, remarkably – and apparently with the help of a seal pushing him to the water's surface – Kevin survived.

From that day onward, it has been Hines's mission to tell his story in the hope that it can help even one person stay alive. His message is to check in on those who seem upset or disturbed.

There's no need for judgement or to try to fix things, other than to simply recognise when another human being is struggling. This is the kind of hope I also intend to carry throughout my life: the hope that there are always opportunities to offer a kind word, a smile, an embrace, a hand, without fear of someone else's mental health problems. It's normal to experience lows and not one of us goes through life unscathed from certain down times, darkness, loss, confusion, turmoil and hardships. It only takes a split second for somebody to lose their precious life – a 'bad' decision by a good person.

Do I want to be a worrier or warrior?

This thought randomly struck me, a few years after losing Scott. I'd gone through the expected patterns of grief as one who had lost her dearest – enduring the first year where every day, event, public holiday or anniversary spurs another reason to reflect, wish longingly, and feel the loss and sadness most powerfully.

It had seemed wicked of life to have me blossoming with a baby on the outside – Scott's baby, the essence of his and my spirit – yet on the inside I felt destroyed and unsure about the road ahead. My ability to grow our baby while also carrying my own sadness, and the prospect of labour minus Scott by my side, was weighing on me. Life felt unsafe and cruel.

I'd already been a single mother and knew acutely how hard that road was, and I was heading into that identity again. Despite this emotional load, I also knew I had to focus on those few things under my control.

It was a lifeline having a son to look forward to – my little version of Scott, whom I suspected would bring us all much joy and distraction from the pain of losing his dad. That's what got me through each day without giving up, as I headed closer to the baby's due date.

Have you experienced a dark night of the soul?

This is when things feel bleak and you're stuck in a state of being that appears to have shut out any light and joy. Blaming someone else, the event or yourself may destroy you. Massive action is the cure all for these moments, and yet sometimes such forward movement feels insurmountable and impossible. Some of my clients have truly believed they would never recover from a loss or something that has affected them to the core. For me too, each day felt like a journey up a mountain.

And yet, if we believe the words of motivational speaker Tony Robbins, we all have the ability to transcend things. He calls this 'post-traumatic growth'. He insists that, in relation to your own healing, it's best to:

- see it as it is, not worse than it is
- see it better than it is
- make it the way you see it.[67]

I can attest to this sentiment. After Liam was born, there were many bittersweet moments, which continue to this day – the fact his hands and feet are just like his dad's and that he is kind of heart, tall and fair, gentle of spirit ... so many genetic traits. I could destroy myself by continuing to harp on with empty feelings of what could have been, or I could choose to see the gifts of our lives, the many precious blessings, that always seem clearer after experiencing a loved one's death.

As a suicide 'widow' with two children, for a while my greatest fear was being alone forever. And yet that worrying energy began to reveal its detriments to me. After a few years of bereavement, I knew that the thing I so desperately sought could only ever be in my grasp if I believed this to be already so, instead of focusing on what I lacked. Three years after losing Scott, I tentatively began to believe that a new future was possible for my family. That I wouldn't be alone in raising children or bereft of the joys of raising my offspring with another devoted adult by my side. I wanted my children to enjoy the sense that they didn't only have me as their guardian in life, or to fear that I could die too and for them to be entirely parent-less. For their lives to be 'normal' would be magic in itself – surely that wasn't too much to dream of, and hope for?

Six months later, not without some initial discomfort and hesitation, I came upon a new loving relationship with a man who, at the time, was incidentally living only a couple of kilometres from our home. It was a slow and measured flow of getting to know each other, of us both working with my bereavement, and becoming slowly but surely committed to each other while honouring Scott's memory. Some years onward and my new partner has taken a step-father role for my daughter Kayli and has happily joined with Liam (after a gradual and sometimes reluctant response from the little man of the house!). Our boy understands his own Dada is in heaven, but he now has another dad 'on earth' to care for him too. I now have the family life I feared would never be ours to enjoy, albeit coloured by our unique experiences.

Liam has asked many times about how Dada got sick and left his body. Answering these tough questions doesn't become easier, nor is there necessarily a 'happily ever after' end to grief – at least not in my realm. As humans, we all experience loss and I believe the journey of living with those cracks in our heart gives meaning to our own lives. I choose to see this as a gift of perspective.

12.

Your Genetics And Constitutional Tendencies

Knowledge is power. You wouldn't embark on a journey in unfamiliar territory without referring to a map – unless you're the kind to 'wing it'. Even then, there is virtue to being pre-warned and having a guide for navigation. And so it is with your body. We all come with predisposing tendencies which can influence our behaviour and life path that are handy to understand, if given the chance.

When new clients arrive at my clinic, part of the consultation experience is about learning what their constitutional and physiological strengths and weaknesses are. We do this with in-depth case taking, exploring family medical history and investigating any existing health records. You may tend toward being diabetic or arthritic due to familial history and if this is the reality, being forewarned means being forearmed, enabling insight to prevent such tendencies playing out.

While most of us are well aware of genetics, you may not have heard of the term nutrigenomics.

※

Nutrigenomics: the genome–food interface

An explanation by Nathaniel Mead in *Environmental Health Perspectives*:

> Although genes are critical for determining function, nutrition modifies the extent to which different genes are expressed and thereby modulates whether individuals attain the potential established by their genetic background. Nutrigenomics therefore initially referred to the study of the effects of nutrients on the expression of an individual's genetic makeup. More recently, this definition has been broadened to encompass nutritional factors that protect the genome from damage. Ultimately, nutrigenomics is concerned with the impact of dietary components on the genome, the proteome (the sum total of all proteins), and the metabolome (the sum of all metabolites).[68]

My interest lies in the interaction of nutrition and genes, especially regarding prevention and/or treatment of disease. The vast options of testing methods available to us now are impressive opening up a great deal of information to quantify and gauge your health status. It means that we're able to blend science with nature – bringing two worlds together for the best outcomes. It's your health, your choice, and however you want to go about securing wellbeing, the tools are at your fingertips. This is a blessing that we enjoy in Australia.

But when does such information become too much? Natural health practitioners are often passionately over-educated as they have a great desire to help their patients. Yet even for them, understanding how these highly complex biochemical processes work for each individual can be overwhelming.

One of the irreplaceable benefits of sitting with a qualified health practitioner is the good old-fashioned virtue of person-to-person assessment. We can observe the way you hold yourself (posture, movement, breathing, speech, demeanour, etc.) when together in clinic. We may feel the warmth or cold clamminess of your hands, or notice the small strands of hair falling on the floor, as you rub and scratch your scalp while we're talking – observations perhaps missed if we're rushing, focused on our computer, typing notes, prematurely moving on to the next consult.

We can witness your tears as you share a story about a loss that correlates with a health condition. We're able to look into your eyes with our iris torches and inspect your fingernails, tongue, skin pallor, and so much more through good old-fashioned case taking, as you sit with us, sometimes for an hour or more, during an initial consultation in our clinic. There's value in this, just as much as there is in me analysing your full blood examination results after I've seen you, looking for more clues as to why, for example, your thyroid is over-functioning.

Dry, cold, hard facts are not enough. Humanising health has and always will be a vital part of the wellness spectrum. Think of the nurse with a 'cold bedside manner' versus a warm and engaged health care provider and you see my point. This is not to say that you cannot get well by self-prescribing in certain cases, but when that's no longer working for you, unravelling the drivers to your unique set of circumstances is most likely to give you the results you've long sought.

Back to nutrigenomics

Numerous studies in humans, animals and cell cultures have demonstrated that macronutrients (e.g. fatty acids and proteins), micronutrients (e.g. vitamins), and naturally occurring bio-reactive chemicals (e.g. phytochemicals such as flavonoids, carotenoids, coumarins, phytosterols and zoochemicals) regulate gene expression in diverse ways. Many of the micronutrients and bio-reactive chemicals in foods are directly involved in metabolic reactions that determine everything from hormonal balances and immune system competence to detoxification processes and the utilisation of macronutrients for fuel and growth.[69]

We all understand that by supplementing our diet, we can achieve positive outcomes. Food as medicine! In Australia, we're fortunate to have such a huge array of wonderful retail products available to us, whether through shopping online or going to our local pharmacy and supplements store. Nevertheless, sometimes we could be working against other factors that influence our body's systems, without realising this is happening. For instance, by wearing certain fabrics or sitting on particular plastics and synthetics, these chemical elements could be disrupting our hormone balance, overriding or detracting from our great vitamin regimen.

To try to make some sense of what's happening with their individual bodies, many of my clients ask for certain testing – be it a salivary hormonal profile, stool or urine test to check for potential deficiencies or pathogens. Then, armed with this information, we can instigate a treatment protocol that includes certain key active constituents and nutrients to either allay any disrupting forces, or to help rebuild, with the aim of these nutrients positively impacting genetic influences.

One step further

Genes aren't straightforward. DNA sequence variations account for 90% of all human genetic variation. These polymorphisms (otherwise known as SNPs) alter the function of 'housekeeping genes' involved in the basic maintenance of the cell, and are assumed to alter the risk of developing a disease. Dietary factors may differentially alter the effect of one or more SNPs to increase or decrease disease risk.

An example of a diet–SNP interaction involves the MTHFR gene.[70] Due to an increase in people undergoing genetic testing of late, shifts in methylation status have gained a great deal of focus.

The key point is that any risks associated with gene activity can be markedly modified, for better or for worse, depending on supplementation strategies – explaining why nutrigenomics is such a fascinating and alluring topic as our technology improves, giving us access to this information.

Nervous system, blood cell health and methylation

Sandra is one of those clients who, like many others, obtained genetic testing; through these results, she was able to ascertain that she has a genetic polymorphism in her body's methylation processes. This impacts the metabolism of key nutrients, with certain health implications such as higher levels of emotional sensitivity, lower energy levels, a greater likelihood of chemical and food sensitivities, body pain and dryness.

The virtue of identifying our genetic history and blueprint is significant. Nonetheless, sometimes too much information can cause confusion and overwhelm, especially when methylation itself is only a tiny aspect of endless other intricate processes happening within the body.

With Sandra, we were able to support her individually, being armed with the insights of her greater health picture. We qualified this with health screening devices and other measures to gauge how her body responded to any treatments she takes. For instance, taking vitamin B12 as an oral sublingual tablet didn't appear to help her much.

However, when we swapped Sandra over to a liposome-delivered B12 (a liquid variety made with sound frequency technology, allowing the remedy to bypass the digestive process to be assimilated into the cell71), her energy levels and red blood cell health improved considerably – something we were able to quantify with tests and more case taking. This highlights that not only method, but delivery is another aspect of success with treatment protocols.

If we choose to follow any kind of dietary regimen, we ought to arm ourselves with the tools to support our body in its own unique way. Sandra invested time and money to see me, to ensure she did things 'right' for her personal make-up. And yet, she also drew on personal intuition when called for. At one point of her training schedule, she was suffering from extreme exhaustion; as a last resort, Sandra sought an iron infusion from her doctor to replenish her system (because she literally couldn't get out of bed due to fatigue). She is not alone in doing this, as several of my clients have found themselves in this situation too. While an iron infusion is useful and sometimes urgently necessary, for Sandra it wasn't the final solution, given that the underlying cause remained.

When I suggested that she could adjust her ideals a little and begin taking a vegetarian (not vegan) therapeutic-grade iron supplement to resolve her imbalance, Sandra agreed. I had confidence this remedy type would help improve her cellular uptake of the mineral, overcoming any chance of biofilm-disrupting agents (for example, an opportunistic pathogen compromising her nutrient stores).

Thankfully, these are the results Sandra enjoyed, and may not have occurred with a lesser quality formula; iron, like most other minerals, needs co-factors for optimal absorption, which we ensured in order to deliver the desired outcome.

After enduring extreme exhaustion and the subsequent frustration of being debilitated over a long timeframe, this improvement was ground breaking for Sandra. She didn't always feel perfect afterwards, but reports to me now that her life has changed because she's no longer afraid of falling back into extreme fatigue, knowing what she needs to stay in her own optimal zone.

As always, you get what you put into life (and yourself). Lasting wellness calls for conscious effort and sometimes for strategic, determined adjustments. Allowing your body to be your teacher is arguably part of the overall process.

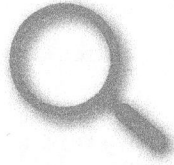

Conclusion

I'm still learning from my body's subtle and not-so-subtle messages.

Acting on these messages while they're still whispers is my aim. Another goal is to not let myself get in the way of this dialogue, given our thoughts are powerful and play their part, not only in our wellbeing, but in what we can achieve and the life we experience.

Dr Christine Page MD, a pioneering holistic doctor whose podcasts I listen to eagerly, believes that 'illness is not a weakness or failure, it's a message from the soul, that can be seen as a soul-ution, instead of a problem'. And most importantly, she reminds us in her many interviews how your body is not affected by physical abuse, but mental abuse. According to her, your mind/thoughts/ emotions can be just as damaging (or conversely healing) as poor dietary habits.'[72]

During a work conference I attended our group of co-workers enjoyed a presentation by a motivational speaker who was introduced as a wise Japanese martial arts and Zen expert. He had the 125 participants engage in group work that demonstrated clearly how the mind can lead the body. The premise was that if you focus on a solution, there is no problem. Conversely, if your mind is ruminating on the problem, then this focus effectively plays out as a blockage.

This was proven to us by two volunteers bravely attempting to break a piece of wood with their hand. The volunteer who was worrying about how to snap the plank, fearful of injuring his hand (i.e. focusing on the 'problem') repeatedly failed to break the plank into two. However, for the woman who focused on the floor, where she expected that piece of wood to land after the blow, her success was immediate. Remarkable!

The presenter reiterated this truth with several other exercises, each with increasing danger or perceived risk. The outcome was always the same! He later shared stories on real cases where his clients overcame their personal limitations or blockages with mindset. The bigger the challenge and crisis, the bigger the opportunity, he pointed out.

Could your symptoms be worth something? Could your focus change the outcome for a particular challenge?

Of course, any of us can be blind-sided with misfortune – loss that doesn't seem fair, or illness that fails to respond to our best efforts of remedy and repair. Whatever the circumstances, it always comes back to the things we can control ourselves – the tools within our immediate power. By tuning into our aches and pains, listening to them and acting on them, we may gather a few gems of wisdom that other outside factors can't teach us. And even though our automatic response may be to push any discomfort away, by surrendering or allowing things to surface, facing them, we might discover unexpected solutions.

As Emma, the late cancer fighter, knew and practiced:

> We are never victims, no matter how hard times may get … For some of us, there is a very particular lesson or message that an illness offers.[73]

> We can approach our recovery motivated by the joy of living or by the fear of dying'. 'The key is to see your disease (or condition) as feedback from your body'.[74]

In his book *I Can See Clearly Now*, the late Dr Wayne Dyer stated 'the mind–body connection is the core of successful self-healing'. Lasting good health may not be a simple case of mind over matter, but our thoughts and responses to illness play a major part in the whole process.[75]

Oprah Winfrey overcame personal trauma to be one of the most influential woman in the US and worldwide. Here is an extract from *What I Know For Sure* that supports her own discovery that your body is your teacher:

> I stopped taking my heart for granted and began thanking it for every beat it had ever given me. I marvelled at the wonder of it: in my 47 years, I'd never consciously given a thought to what my heart does, feeding oxygen to my lungs, liver, pancreas, even my brain, one beat at a time.

> For so many years, I had let my heart down by not giving it the support it needed. Overeating. Over-stressing. Overdoing. No wonder when I lay down at night it couldn't stop racing. I believe everything that happens in our lives

has meaning, that each experience brings a message, if we're willing to hear it. So what was my speeding heart trying to tell me? I still didn't know the answer. Yet simply asking the question caused me to look at my body and how I had failed to honour it. Taking care of my heart, the life force of my body, had never been my priority.

I sat up in bed one crisp, sunny morning and made a vow to love my heart. To treat it with respect. To feed and nurture it. To work it out and then let it rest.

… What I know for sure: there is no need to struggle with your body when you make a loving and grateful peace with it.'[76]

Likewise, I encourage you to explore the possibility that your thoughts and feelings could be playing a part in your symptoms; notice the times when this might be occurring for you. It's been impressive and a privilege to witness my clients, over the years, overcoming a sense of sickness by drawing on not only naturopathic support, but also their own inner resolve to make that happen.

Remember that wellbeing is the dominant order of life, and when we find ourselves stuck in a condition, we need to try to move from any sense of overwhelm to hopefulness. It takes a leap of faith, but it's a vital part of healing, and of nurturing ourselves.

Dr Bruce Lipton, author of *The Biology of Belief*, notes that around 70% of our thoughts are negative or redundant. Our self-talk can be our downfall or our saviour. He reminds us that fire-walkers are able to complete a physically dangerous feat by talking themselves into believing that the fire will not harm or burn them. Likewise, the Pentecostal Baptists from southern USA, who drink poisonous vapour and endure deadly snake venom, sustain their lives by working themselves into such an elevated mental state that this fervour manages to protect them from physical realities.[77]

While I'm not radical enough to push the envelope that far, having a good hold on self-preservation and comfort, I *am* committed to listening to my body and continuously exploring the space between what is vs what can be. I'm grateful for all the victories achieved and recoveries we've made – being able to walk again after the threat of paralysis, revitalising after fatigue and birthing two healthy babies, despite also losing one before it reached life. All the little triumphs after so many health crises and setbacks, which will no doubt keep presenting in my life, allowed me to hone in on what needs my attention.

To end, a poem by Kate Ellis, the remarkable teacher and writer:

Thank you for keeping me here

Earth

Thank you for telling me what feels wrong

And what is so very right

Body.[78]

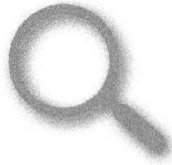

Acknowledgements

To James Hardiman, thank you for backing my every pursuit and for your unconditional love. And to my late beloved Scott Pittaway and his family for their kinship and support, making it possible to bring Liam into the world, raising him as a happy, healthy boy.

To my aunty Bernie O'Connell and sister Fiona O'Connell, your constructive input is highly valued, as always. Thank you to my parents Liisa and Kerry, who allowed me the length of rope to explore life so fully, always nourishing our family and me. *Kiitos* to my Finnish Aunt Helena, who first ignited the 'health freak' part of my soul. My late grandmother Gabrielle O'Connell, who suffered mental illness and institutionalisation: your spiritual purpose, despite difficult social times and personal hardships, continues to inspire me in the field of mental health, as a fellow mother, woman and self-growth seeker. I still feel your loving presence, Nana, just like those times together when I was a little girl.

To Busybird Publishing, my gratitude for your expertise, particularly that of editor Beau Hillier for being so thorough.

And to all naturopaths in our country, I humbly applaud you. Ours is not an easy profession to succeed and flourish in. Your big-heartedness and efforts have vital impact. I feel blessed and buoyed to work beside and with a body of dedicated and highly educated practitioners, who continue to balance the scales of our increasingly sick society.

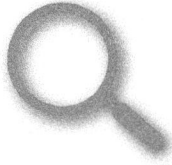

About The Author

*J*ulie is a long-accredited Australian Naturopath and Herbalist with a career history in Marketing, Writing and Publishing.

She has a clinical practice in Melbourne where she facilitates healthy body support groups.

Also a Trainer for a leading Australian supplements range, Julie educates Pharmacists and their staff on safe and effective methods in supporting consumer's best health outcomes.

A mother of two and passionate advocate for the destigmatisation of mental illness, Julie continues to strive in making a difference through the natural health arena.

Read her blog and find reader special offers

@

www.julieseamer.com.au.

If you have enjoyed this book discover more interesting case studies and connect with other readers
@

www.yourbodyisyourteacher.com

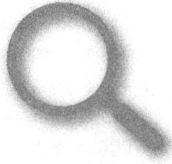

Endnotes

1 Heim, E 1980, *Illness as Crisis and Opportunity*

2 Dethlefsen, T; Dahlke, R & Lemesurier, P 1997, *The Healing Power of Illness: Understanding what your symptoms are telling you*, Element Books, Australia, p. 72

3 Mars, M 2018, 'The Suffering of the soul in medicine: Psychosomatic medicine, depression, anxiety, anger and the skin', *Journal of The Australian Traditional Medicine Society*, Vol. 24, No. 1, pp. 8–11. And: Furst, L 2003, *Idioms of distress: Psychosomatic disorders in medical and imaginative literature*, State University of New York Press: New York.

4 Dethlefsen, T; Dahlke, R & Lemesurier, P, op cit., p. 81

5 Poole, G c.f., 'Male suicides in Australia up 10 per cent in 2017', AMHF, <https://www.amhf.org.au/male_suicides_in_australia_up_10_in_2017>

6 Noontil, A 1994, *The Body is the Barometer of the Soul*, Brumby Books

7 Elshemy, A & Abobakr, M 2013, 'Allergic Reaction: Symptoms, Diagnosis, Treatment and Management', Department of Pharmacy, International Islamic University Chittagong, Chittagong, Bangladesh, Journal of Scientific & Innovative Research, Vol. 2, No. 1, p. 123, <http://www.jsirjournal.com/Vol2Issue1013.pdf>

8 Ford, R 2011, 'Food allergy causes eczema', The Children's Clinic and The Allergy Centre, <https://www.thechildrensclinic.co.nz/eczema/food-allergy>

9 'The Link Between Food Tolerance and Eczema', ImuPro, <https://imupro.com.au/link-food-intolerance-eczema/>

10 Pang, G et al. 2012, 'How functional foods play critical roles in human health', *Food Science and Human Wellness*, Vol. 1, No. 1, pp. 26–60, <https://www.sciencedirect.com/science/article/pii/S2213453012000055>

11 Bilski, J et al. 2017, 'The Role of Intestinal Alkaline Phosphatase in Inflammatory Disorders of Gastrointestinal Tract', <https://www.ncbi.nlm.nih.gov/pubmed/28316376>. And: Estaki, M et al. 2014, 'Interplay between intestinal alkaline phosphatase, diet, gut microbes and immunity', *World Journal of Gastroenterology*, Vol. 20, No. 42, <https://www.ncbi.nlm.nih.gov/pmc/articles/PMC4229529/>

12 Augusti, A et al. 2018, 'Interplay Between the Gut-Brain Axis, Obesity and Cognitive Function', *Frontiers in Neuroscience*, Vol. 12, <https://www.ncbi.nlm.nih.gov/pmc/articles/PMC5864897/>. And: Liang, S et al. 2018, 'Gut-Brain Psychology: Rethinking Psychology From the Microbiota–Gut–Brain Axis', *Frontiers in Integrative Neuroscience*, Vol. 12, <https://www.ncbi.nlm.nih.gov/pmc/articles/PMC6142822/>

13 Bowe, Whitney & Logan, Alan 2011, 'Acne vulgaris, probiotics and the gut-brain-skin axis – back to the future?', *Gut Pathogens*, Vol. 3, No. 1, <https://www.ncbi.nlm.nih.gov/pmc/articles/PMC3038963/>

14 ibid.

15 ibid.

16 'What is GBS?', The Guillain–Barré Syndrome Association of NSW, <http://www.gbs-cidp-nsw.org.au/information/what-is-gbs?showall=1&limitstart=>

17 Novak, M & Vetvicka, V 2007, 'β-Glucans, History, and the Present: Immunomodulatory Aspects and Mechanisms of Action', *Journal of Immunotoxicology*, Vol. 5, No. 1, pp. 47–57, <http://doi.org/10.1080/15476910802019045>; Soltanian, S et al. 2009, 'Beta-glucans as immunostimulant in vertebrates and invertebrates', *Critical Reviews in Microbiology*, Vol. 35, No.2, pp. 109–138.

18 Gao et al. 2003. 'Effects of Ganopoly (A Ganoderma lucidum polysaccharide extract) on the immune functions in advanced-stage cancer patients', *Immunological Investigations*, Vol. 32, No. 3, pp. 201–215; Yoon, TJ, Koppula, S & Lee, KH 2013, 'The effects of β-glucans on cancer metastasis', *Anti-Cancer Agents in Medicinal Chemistry*, Vol. 13, No. 5, pp. 699–708; Yamaguchi et al. 2011, 'Efficacy and safety of orally administered Lentinula edodes mycelia extract for patients undergoing cancer chemotherapy: a pilot study', *The American Journal of Chinese Medicine*, Vol. 39, No. 3, pp. 451–459.

19 'Astragalus benefits', Indigo Herbs, <https://www.indigo-herbs.co.uk/natural-health-guide/benefits/astragalus>

20 Dethlefsen, T; Dahlke, R & Lemesurier, P, op cit., p. 148

21 'Taste and Smell Research' 2017, National Institute on Deafness and Other Communication Disorders, <https://www.nidcd.nih.gov/about/strategic-plan/2017-2021/taste-and-smell-research>

22 Tierra, M, 'Integrating the Traditional Chinese Theory and Treatment of the Lungs with that of Western Physiology', <https://planetherbs.com/research-center/theory-articles/integrating-the-traditional-chinese-theory-and-treatment-of-the-lungs-with-that-of-western-physiology/>

23 Suttie, E 2016, 'Grief and the Lungs', Chinese Medicine Living, <https://www.chinesemedicineliving.com/philosophy/the-emotions/grief-the-lungs/>

24 Lehrer, Paul; Isenberg, Susan & Hochron, Stuart 2009, 'Asthma and Emotion: A Review', *Journal of Asthma*, Vol. 30, pp. 5–21, <https://www.tandfonline.com/doi/abs/10.3109/02770909309066375>

25 Ma, C & Leung, Y 2017, 'Exploring the Link between Uric Acid and Osteoarthritis', <https://doi.org/10.3389/fmed.2017.00225/>

26 Vormann, J et al. 2001, 'Supplementation with alkaline minerals reduces symptoms in patients with chronic low back pain', *Journal of Trace Elements in Medicine and Biology*, Vol. 15, No. 2–3, pp. 179–183, <https://www.sciencedirect.com/science/article/pii/S0946672X0180064X>; Frassetto, L op cit. 2018, 'Acid Balance, Dietary Acid Load, and Bone Effects – A Controversial Subject', *Nutrients*, Vol. 19, No. 4, <https://www.ncbi.nlm.nih.gov/pmc/articles/PMC5946302/>

27 'Arthritis and diet', Better Health Channel, Department of Health & Human Services, State Government of Victoria, <https://www.betterhealth.vic.gov.au/health/conditionsandtreatments/arthritis-and-diet>

28 Vormann, J et al., op cit.

29 Ng, QX et al. 2017, 'Clinical Use of Curcumin in Depression: A Meta-Analysis', Journal of the American Medical Director's Association, Vol. 18, No. 6, pp. 503–508, <https://www.ncbi.nlm.nih.gov/pubmed/28236605>

30 Uziel, Y & Hashkes, P 2007, 'Growing pains in children', *Pediatric Rheumatology*, <https://ped-rheum.biomedcentral.com/articles/10.1186/1546-0096-5-5>.

31 Man, K et al. 2016, 'Methylphenidate and the risk of psychotic disorders and hallucinations in children and adolescents in a large health system', *Translational Psychiatry*, Vol. 6, No. 11, <https://www.ncbi.nlm.nih.gov/pmc/articles/PMC5314128/>

32 Kamper, S et al. 2016, 'Musculoskeletal pain in children and adolescents', *Brazilian Journal of Physical Therapy*, Vol. 20, No. 3, pp. 275–284, <https://www.ncbi.nlm.nih.gov/pmc/articles/PMC4946844/>.

33 Shetty. S et al. 2016, 'Bone turnover markers: Emerging tool in the management of osteoporosis', *Indian Journal of Endocrinology and Metabolism*, Vol. 20, No. 6, pp. 846–852, <https://www.ncbi.nlm.nih.gov/pmc/articles/PMC5105571/>

34 Rössler, W 2016, 'The stigma of mental disorders: A millennia-long history of social exclusion and prejudices', *EMBO Reports*, Vol. 17, No. 9, pp. 1250–1253, <https://www.ncbi.nlm.nih.gov/pmc/articles/PMC5007563/>

35 Volkow, N 2012, 'The genetics of addiction', HHS Author Manuscripts, Vol. 131, No. 6, pp. 773–777, <https://www.ncbi.nlm.nih.gov/pmc/articles/PMC4101188/>

36 .Ducci, F & Goldman, D 2012, 'The Genetic Basis of Addictive Disorders', HHS Author Manuscripts, Psychiatric Clinic of North America, Vol. 35, No. 2, pp. 495–519, <https://www.ncbi.nlm.nih.gov/pmc/articles/PMC3506170/>

37 Lu, S 2009, 'Regulation of glutathione synthesis', *Molecular Aspects of Medicine*, Vol. 30, No. 1–2, pp. 42–59, <https://www.ncbi.nlm.nih.gov/pubmed/18601945/#>

38 MacLeod, C 2013, 'N-acetyl-cysteine: A Versatile Intervention', *Integrapted Healthcare Practitioners*, <http://ihpmagazine.com/n-acetyl-cysteine-a-versatile-intervention/>

39 Lavoie, S et al. 2008, 'Glutathione precursor, N-acetyl-cysteine, improves mismatch negativity in schizophrenia patients', *Neuropsychopharmacology*, Vol. 33, No. 9, pp. 2187–99, <https://www.ncbi.nlm.nih.gov/pubmed/18004285>.

40 De Rosa, SC et al. 2000, 'N-acetylcysteine replenishes glutathione in HIV infection', *European Journal of Clinical Investigation*, Vol. 30, No. 10, pp. 915–29, <https://www.ncbi.nlm.nih.gov/pubmed/11029607>.

41 Chen, CH & Young, YH 2017, 'N-acetylcysteine as a single therapy for sudden deafness', *Acta Oto-laryngologica*, Vol. 137, No. 1, pp. 58–62, <https://www.ncbi.nlm.nih.gov/pubmed/27553486>

42 Thakker, D et al. 2015, 'N-Acetylcysteine for Polycystic Ovary Syndrome: A Systematic Review and Meta-Analysis of Randomized Controlled Clinical Trials', *Obstetrics and Gynecology International*, <https://www.ncbi.nlm.nih.gov/pmc/articles/PMC4306416/>

43 Dethlefsen op cit., p. 103

44 Anunike, KC 2015, 'Coping With Injury: How High-Performance Athletes Mitigate the Biopsychosocial Consequences of Sports Injury', Psychiatry and Behavioural Sciences, Master's thesis, Duke University, p. 20, <http://hdl.handle.net/10161/15736>

45 Stewart, K 2018, private interview with Julie O'Connell-Seamer.

46 Anunike, KC op cit., p. 25. And: Tesarz, J et al. 2012, 'Pain perception in athletes compared to normally active controls: a systematic review with meta-analysis', *Pain*, Vol. 153, No. 6, pp. 1253–62, <https://www.ncbi.nlm.nih.gov/pubmed/22607985>

47 ibid, p. 22

48 Stoltz, P & Weihenmayer, E 2008, The Adversity Advantage: Turning Everyday Struggles Into Everyday Greatness, Simon & Schuster, p. xvii.

49 Pasco, J et al. 2014, 'Body mass index and measures of body fat for defining obesity and underweight: a cross-sectional, population-based study', *BMC Obesity*, <https://www.ncbi. nlm.nih.gov/pmc/articles/PMC4511447>

50 Sansone, R & Sansone, L 2011, 'Personality Pathology and Its Influence on Eating Disorders', *Innovations in Clinical Neuroscience*, Vol. 8, No. 3, pp. 14–18, <https://www.ncbi.nlm. nih.gov/pmc/articles/PMC3074200/>

51 'Anorexia nervosa', Better Health Channel, Department of Health & Human Services, State Government of Victoria, <https://www.betterhealth.vic.gov.au/health/healthyliving/anorexia-nervosa>

52 Buckner, CA et al. 2018, 'Complementary and alternative medicine use in patients before and after a cancer diagnosis', *Current Oncology*, Vol. 25, No. 4, pp. e275–e281, <https:// www.ncbi.nlm.nih.gov/pmc/articles/PMC6092049/>

53 vanderHoeven, E, *Diagnosis to Recovery: The Path to Wholeness,* a guide to conscious health care through mindset, Busybird Publishing, p. 25

54 ibid, p. 22

55 ibid, pp. 21–2

56 ibid, pp. 41–2

57 ibid, p. 12

58 ibid, p. 18

59 ibid, p. 34

60 ibid, p. 35

61 ibid, p. 48

62 ibid, p. 55

63 ibid, p. 56

64 ibid

65 Röing, M & Sanner, M 2015, 'A meta-ethnographic synthesis on phenomenographic studies of patients' experiences of chronic illness', *International Journal of Qualitative Studies on Health and Well-being*, Vol. 10, No. 1, <https://doi.org/10.3402/qhw.v10.26279>

66 Marton, F; Bowden, JA & Walsh, E 2000, 'The structure of awareness', *Phenomenography,* Melbourne: RMIT University Press. p. 105

67 Robbins, T, 'Reframing Post-Traumatic Growth', <https://www.tonyrobbins.com/personal-growth/reframing-posttraumatic-growth/>

68 Mead, N 2007, 'Nutrigenomics: The Genome–Food Interface', *Environmental Health Perspectives*, Vol. 115, No. 12, pp. A582–A589, <https://www.ncbi.nlm.nih.gov/pmc/articles/ PMC2137135/>

69 ibid; Pang, G et al., op. cit.; Skenkin, A 2006, 'Micronutrients in health and disease', Postgraduate Medical Journal, Vol. 82, No. 971, pp. 559–567, <https://www.ncbi.nlm.nih.gov/pmc/ articles/PMC2585731/>; Faria, AMC et al. 2013, 'Food Components and the Immune System: From Tonic Agents to Allergens', Frontiers in Immunology, Vol. 4, <https://www.ncbi.nlm.nih. gov/pmc/articles/PMC3656403/>

70 'What is MTHFR?', MTHFRSupport, <https://www.mthfrsupport.com.au/what-is-mthfr/>

71 Keller, BC 2001, 'Liposomes in Nutrition', *Trends in Food Science and Technology* Vol. 12, pp. 25–31.

72 Page, C, 'Dr Christine Page', *In Short Order* (podcast), <http://www.blogtalkradio.com/in-short-order/2016/11/17/in-short-order--dr-christine-page>, Frontiers of Health, <https://www.christinepage.com/offerings/wellness/the-gift-of-illness/>

73 vanderHoeven, E op cit., p. 72

74 ibid, p. 84

75 Dyer, W 2014, *I Can See Clearly Now*, Dr Wayne Dyer, Hay House, pp. 73-4

76 Winfrey, O 2014, *What I Know For Sure*, Macmillan, NY, USA

77 Lipton, B 2005, *The Biology of Belief*, Hay House

78 Ellis, K, <https://www.kateelliscoaching.com/>

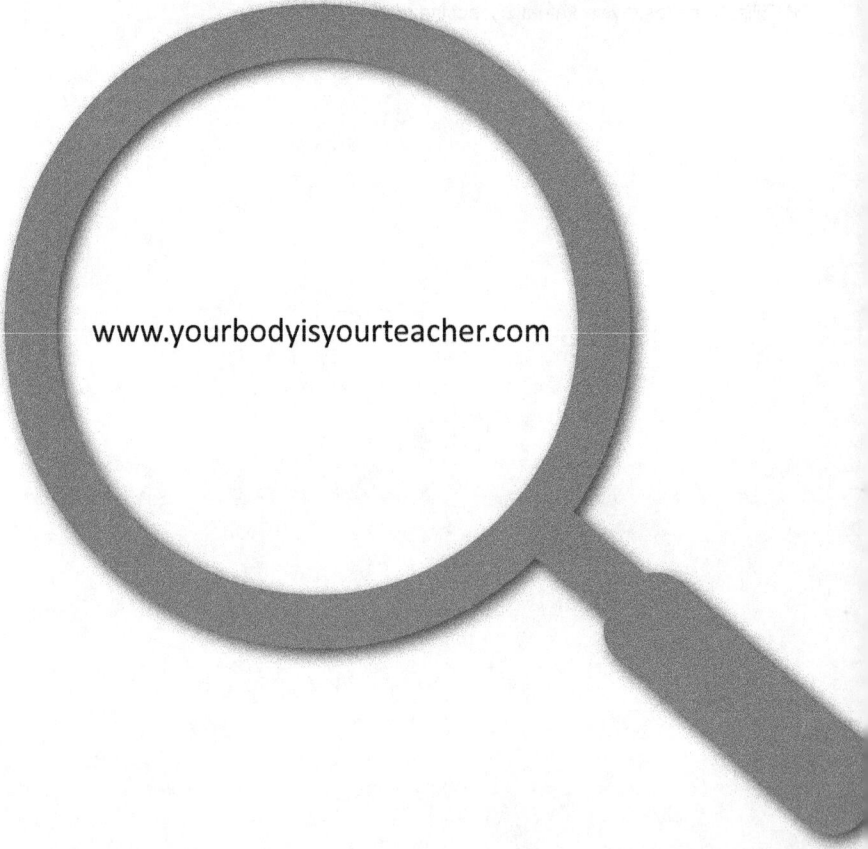

www.yourbodyisyourteacher.com

www.ingramcontent.com/pod-product-compliance
Lightning Source LLC
Chambersburg PA
CBHW021831020426
42334CB00014B/578